The
COMPLETE VEGAN
AIR FRYER
COOKBOOK

150 PLANT-BASED RECIPES
FOR YOUR FAVORITE FOODS

SUSAN LABORDE *and* ELIZABETH HICKMAN

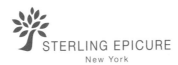

STERLING EPICURE
New York

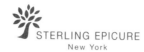

STERLING EPICURE
New York

An Imprint of Sterling Publishing Co., Inc.
1166 Avenue of the Americas
New York, NY 10036

ISBN 978-1-4549-3310-6

Distributed in Canada by Sterling Publishing Co., Inc.
c/o Canadian Manda Group, 664 Annette Street
Toronto, Ontario, M6S 2C8, Canada
Distributed in the United Kingdom by GMC Distribution Services
Castle Place, 166 High Street, Lewes, East Sussex, BN7 1XU, United Kingdom
Distributed in Australia by NewSouth Books
University of New South Wales, Sydney, NSW 2052, Australia

For information about custom editions,
special sales, and premium and corporate purchases,
please contact Sterling Special Sales at
800-805-5489 or specialsales@sterlingpublishing.com.

Manufactured in Canada

2 4 6 8 10 9 7 5 3 1

sterlingpublishing.com

Interior design by Gavin Motnyk
Cover design by David Ter-Avanesyan
based on an original design by Elizabeth Mihaltse Lindy
Food Styling by Dianne Vezza

For image credits, see page 176.

CONTENTS

INTRODUCTION

Welcome to the wonderful world of air frying! If you think this odd-looking appliance is just an expensive French fry machine, you're in for lots of delicious surprises. Of course we understand if you're skeptical. We were born and raised in the Deep South, where fried food is king and virtually every food is fried. Imagine trying to get that great fried taste without all the grease. It's impossible—or so we thought.

As soon as we started using one, we realized that air fryers do indeed work. Perhaps most amazing is that, with some foods such as fresh okra (page 36) and mushrooms (page 10), the air-fryer version is *better* than deep-fried. What a pleasure to be able to enjoy the fried foods we love without consuming so much oil. The appliance spares you from the huge mess of deep frying because you use only minimal amounts of oil—which means no big pot of grease to spatter all over your range and countertop—and it helps you make food with fewer calories and less guilt.

Air fryers are incredibly versatile. In these pages, you'll discover a full range of dishes for every time of day. For starters, you can enjoy healthier versions of all your favorite fried foods, but there's so much more. You can cook asparagus (page 79), eggplant (page 31), and so many other vegetables quickly and with delicious results. Also check out the recipes for muffins and breads. Baked goods (page 121) turn out beautifully.

Air fryers aren't complicated, but they do take a little getting used to because the cooking method itself is unique. Start with something simple such as French Fries (page 91) or Roasted Nuts (page 39). Once you have some experience, we hope you'll use this cookbook as a springboard for developing your own new favorites. Many of our recipes suggest variations, and we hope those will trigger other ideas for you to test and enjoy.

Over time, you may find yourself using your air fryer every day—and that wouldn't surprise us. It offers so many advantages. It's fast and convenient and works well on almost everything. It doesn't make a big mess, it's easy to clean, and on sweltering summer days it doesn't heat up your kitchen like an oven does.

We had great fun creating our first cookbook, *The Air Fryer Bible*, and we're pleased to offer this collection of recipes—all of them tested in our home kitchens—developed especially for you, our vegan friends. We sincerely hope that this cookbook helps you make the most of your air fryer, a fun and unique way to cook healthier!

TIPS FOR SUCCESS

Read the Manual

Almost everyone hates reading instruction manuals, but it won't take long, and, trust us, it's time well spent. There are dozens of air fryer brands and models available, and no two are identical. Features, functions, and even construction materials can differ greatly, all of which affect appliance use and care. **Read all safety information, and never use your air fryer in any way that violates the manufacturer's instructions for safe use.**

Your manual should include information about other serious concerns, such as protecting your kitchen surfaces and allowing for sufficient ventilation around the back, sides, and top of your appliance. Note that, in addition to potential safety risks, any misuse of your air fryer or its parts could void the manufacturer's warranty.

Cooking Time

All recipes in this cookbook were tested in 1,425-watt air fryers with standard capacity—*not* extra-large size. We've found that some air fryers cook more slowly than others, especially the more inexpensive models. Other factors that can affect cooking times include:

- amount of food in basket or number of layers
- amount or thickness of breading or coating
- size (dimensions) of pieces of food being cooked
- temperature of food when placed in fryer

Even the air temperature or humidity level in your kitchen can make a difference. For best results, we recommend the following:

- Cut foods into uniform pieces for more even cooking.
- When a recipe calls for a single layer, do not stack foods.
- Follow recipe directions to shake basket or stir foods to redistribute during cooking. If your appliance tends to cook unevenly, you may need to shake or stir more often than the recipe indicates.
- **Always begin with the shortest cooking time listed in a recipe.**

That last point is the most important, especially when you're new to air frying or have a brand-new appliance. Avoid overcooking by checking food early and often. The interior of an air fryer reheats very quickly, so don't worry about pausing often to open the drawer.

Cooking in Batches

We used standard-size air fryers for testing all of the recipes developed for this cookbook. These units have an interior capacity of approximately 3 quarts. Many of our recipes call for cooking two batches, which still saves you time because the foods cook so quickly.

When recipes call for longer cooking times,

your first batch may cool before the second finishes. In that case, simply pause your air fryer shortly before the second batch is done and add the first batch for the remaining cooking time. If your basket won't hold the entire recipe, finish the second batch completely, then cook the first batch for a minute or two to reheat.

Air fryers are excellent at reheating, which makes them the perfect solution for all kinds of leftovers. Have you ever tried to reheat French fries? The oven dries them out, and the microwave makes them tough and rubbery. Put them in your air fryer, though, and they will turn out hot, crispy, and much closer to freshly cooked.

If you own a 5-quart (or similar) air fryer, you should be able to cook many of our recipes in one batch. Don't stack or crowd the food unless the recipe allows for that. Begin with the shortest cooking time listed and check often for doneness. With a little experience, you'll get a feel for how much you may need to adjust the cooking time.

Smoking

First, read what your air fryer manufacturer says about smoking. Excessive smoking is *not* normal and could indicate a malfunction. If that happens, safely and immediately disconnect the power from the appliance and contact the manufacturer.

You may experience smoke coming from your air fryer when cooking certain foods. For example, coconut tends to smoke easily. For this reason, you should take care in choosing the location for using the appliance. One of the best places is next to your range so that you can take advantage of its vent hood.

Also, allowing too much oil to accumulate in your air fryer drawer can cause smoke, especially when using oils with a low smoke point. You can prevent this problem by keeping the drawer clean and free of food and excess oil. If you're in the middle of dinner and need to stop the smoke so you can finish cooking, try adding a little water to the air fryer drawer.

TERMS & TECHNIQUES

As we've said, air fryers are simple to operate, but the cooking method itself is unique. If you're getting acquainted with your appliance, we offer the following information to help clarify the most commonly used terms and techniques in our recipes.

Baking Pan

For recipe testing, we always use a 6 x 6 x 3-inch air fryer baking pan. Another common size is 6 inches diameter round by 3 inches deep. You can use oven-safe dishes that fit in your air fryer, but you may find it difficult to remove them from the basket when filled with hot food. You can fashion a makeshift basket from folded aluminum foil, but, for convenience and safety, we much prefer using a pan with a handle made specifically for use in air fryers. Prices for these pans are very reasonable, and it's worth the small investment if you want to enjoy air fryer cooking to the fullest.

Cooking Spray

The convenience of aerosol cooking sprays is very tempting, but they have obvious environmental drawbacks. Wherever possible, we prefer to use a pump-style sprayer or a refillable hand-pumped mister, but sometimes only cooking spray will do, particularly with delicate foods when even extra-light olive oil might add unwanted flavor.

Dredging Station

This is just a simple assembly line for breading foods before frying. It consists of 2 or 3 shallow dishes, each containing a dry or liquid mixture in which to dip your food. For example, you line up cornstarch, almond milk, and breadcrumbs in dredging order, which speeds the coating process. For clarity and convenience, we specify ingredients and order instead of using the term "dredging station."

Gloves

Restaurant supply shops and online stores carry disposable food-grade gloves. Poly or rubber gloves fit loosely and tend to be too stiff. We recommend powder-free, food-grade vinyl or latex, and you should choose a snug fit for maximum flexibility. They're useful for working with hot peppers or any time you have to prep food by hand.

Muffin Cups

Some recipes call for paper or foil muffin cups, sometimes doubled or tripled. The choice depends on the type of filling. Foil cups are stronger and work better with more liquid contents. For more strength, double the foil cups by removing the paper liners, stacking, then misting the interior cup with oil if needed.

Another option is oven-safe silicone muffin cups. We highly recommend them! They hold their shape much better and can support even the most liquid fillings.

Oil for Misting

A pastry brush works in a pinch, but we don't recommended it because brushes add more oil than necessary for air frying. Our first choice is a refillable, pump-style mister. Invest in a good one. It's easy to use and works well whether you need a fine mist or a heavier coating. It's also more environmentally friendly because it doesn't use aerosols, wind up in landfills, or need recycling.

For the oil, we recommend extra-light olive oil because it has a higher smoke point than extra-virgin olive oil and it has an extremely mild taste unnoticeable on most foods (with the exception of certain sweets or delicately flavored dishes).

RECIPE CODES

Most recipes in this book feature the labels or codes listed below. They're self-explanatory, but here are short descriptions for each code.

Fast — 15 minutes or fewer from start to finish

Gluten Free — No proteins from barley, rye, or wheat

Great Snack — Ideal for eating between meals

Kid Friendly — Little ones will love these.

Super Easy — A minimal number of simple steps, perfect for beginners

Taster Favorite — Great for lots of different palates.

At the back of the book (page 168), you'll find a table of all the recipes along with these codes so that you can search quickly for exactly the dish you want.

INGREDIENTS

Definitions and explanations in this section apply throughout the cookbook. This is a vegan cookbook, so we try not to repeat the word in the ingredient lists, but we do use it selectively to avoid confusion. In addition to the specific foods below, every ingredient we list means the vegan version of a particular food.

Breadcrumbs are finely crushed and relatively dry. They may act as a filler or coating to produce a light crust. Use plain, unseasoned breadcrumbs unless a recipe states otherwise, Italian breadcrumbs for example.

    Panko breadcrumbs consist of larger, firmer flakes than traditional breadcrumbs. They're the best choice for maximum crunch. Crushed panko has a slightly different texture better suited to certain foods. You can crush panko in a food processor or by placing the crumbs in a plastic bag and pounding it with a rolling pin.

Dairy, such as butter, cheese, sour cream, and yogurt, always means the non-dairy, certified-vegan versions of these products. We tested all of the recipes in this book using Bob's Red Mill **egg replacer**. All replacers and substitutes *don't* perform the same. Using any other brand in these recipes may produce extremely different results.

Flours vary greatly and aren't always interchangeable. In recipes with no type of flour specified, use plain all-purpose white flour. Bleached, unbleached, or all-purpose flour is refined flour with the bran removed. Manufacturers add nutrients to enrich the flour and compensate for the vitamins and minerals lost in processing. Self-rising flour contains leavening agents added to help baked goods rise. Self-rising flour and plain all-purpose flour are not interchangeable.

Pioneers of the nineteenth century prized white flour for its keeping qualities. White-bread loaves kept longer in larders than whole-wheat loaves. The same holds true today. White flours have a longer shelf life than whole-grain products, but these flours do have their appealing qualities. For high fluffy biscuits, scones, yeast breads, textured cakes, and tender baked goods, only a good white flour will do.

Whole-wheat flour is healthier because it retains the fiber and nutrients of the whole grain. The downside, for some uses, is that the end product can become heavy and dense. We use two types of whole-wheat flour. Most people are familiar with red wheat, which is heartier than enriched flour but can make baked goods heavy and dense—sometimes a good thing. Some recipes use a combination of white flour and whole-wheat to lighten a dough or batter.

Our favorite whole-wheat flour is white wheat. Not the same as white all-purpose flour, it comes from a different strain of wheat and yields a baked good somewhere between a heavy loaf made from red wheat and a light, white-flour loaf. If you can't find white-wheat flour at your local grocery store, it's available online.

Always store whole-wheat flours in a glass jar in the refrigerator.

Garlic powder should contain only one ingredient: garlic. Never substitute garlic salt.

You need to crush dried **herbs and spices** (dill, rosemary, oregano, etc.) to release their natural oils. To crush, measure the amount given in the recipe, then rub the herbs gently between your forefinger and thumb as you allow the herbs to fall onto the food.

How to Measure Crushed Ingredients

Method makes a big difference. When a recipe calls for "1/2 cup crushed [ingredient]," crush *before* measuring. When recipe calls for "1/2 cup [ingredient], crushed," measure before crushing.

Meats, such as bacon, pepperoni, and sausage, always mean the certified-vegan imitation meat products.

We tested all recipes calling for **milk** with unflavored, unsweetened almond milk, unless the recipe states otherwise. We prefer the Diamond brand because it's not overly thick, unlike many other non-dairy milks.

Olive oil offers health benefits as well as great taste. Extra-virgin, first cold-pressed olive oil has a distinctive flavor that can enhance a finished dish. It also can prove overwhelming, especially a robust version. For misting, use a light or extra-light olive oil with the most delicate flavor.

Pepper always means black peppercorns freshly ground.

Salt always means sea salt.

BREAKFAST & BRUNCH

Breakfast Cornbread

Yield: 4 servings | Prep Time: 13 minutes | Cooking Time: 12–13 minutes | Total Time: 25–26 minutes

Southerners can never get enough cornbread. Toasty pecans and a touch of sweetness make this a great way to enjoy this favorite treat for breakfast.

1 tablespoon flaxseed meal

2 tablespoons water

½ cup pecans, roughly chopped

½ cup white cornmeal

½ cup all-purpose white flour

2 teaspoons baking powder

½ teaspoon salt

2 tablespoons vegetable oil

½ cup almond milk

2 tablespoons molasses

maple syrup for serving

1. Preheat the air fryer to 360°F.

2. In a medium bowl, mix the flaxseed meal and water and set aside.

3. Place the pecans in the air fryer baking pan and cook for 2 to 3 minutes, until toasted. Remove from the pan and set aside.

4. In a large bowl, stir together the cornmeal, flour, baking powder, and salt.

5. To the flaxseed mixture, add the oil, milk, and molasses and whisk together.

6. Pour the wet ingredients into the dry ingredients and stir to mix well.

7. Pour the batter into the air fryer baking pan and cook for 12 to 13 minutes or until a toothpick inserted into the center comes out clean.

8. Remove from the air fryer and cool in the pan for 5 minutes.

9. Cut the bread diagonally into 4 wedges.

10. Top with the toasted pecans and maple syrup and serve warm.

See insert A1 for recipe photo.

Coconut Bacon

Yield: 2 cups | Prep Time: 5 minutes | Cooking Time: 7–9 minutes | Total Time: 12–14 minutes

FAST   SUPER EASY   TASTER FAVORITE

Serve this as a side or topping for any breakfast dish. It also adds a flavor boost to sandwiches, salads, potatoes, and other vegetables.

---

oil for misting or cooking spray

2 cups unsweetened, large coconut chips

2 tablespoons low-sodium soy sauce

5 teaspoons liquid smoke

1 tablespoon maple syrup

1. Preheat the air fryer to 360°F.

2. Spray the air fryer baking pan lightly with oil or nonstick spray.

3. Place the coconut chips in the baking pan.

4. In a small bowl, mix the soy sauce, liquid smoke, and syrup.

5. Pour the liquid over the coconut chips and stir well to distribute.

6. Cook for 3 minutes, then stir.

7. Cook for 2 more minutes and stir again.

8. Cook for another 2 minutes and stir a third time.

9. If needed, cook for an additional 1 to 2 minutes, but watch closely to make sure the chips don't burn. It can happen very quickly!

10. Serve hot or spread the chips on a baking sheet to cool slightly. The chips will crisp as they cool.

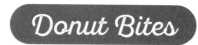

Donut Bites

Yield: 16 bites | Prep Time: 10 minutes | Cooking Time: 4–5 minutes per batch (2 batches) | Total Time: 18–20 minutes

GREAT SNACK   KID FRIENDLY

Tofu gives these sweet treats some protein for staying power, and the air fryer eliminates the need for deep frying these in unhealthy oils.

---

1 tablespoon Bob's Red Mill egg replacer

2 tablespoons water

1 cup all-purpose white flour

4 tablespoons coconut sugar, divided

1 teaspoon baking powder

$1/4$ teaspoon baking soda

$1/8$ teaspoon salt

4 ounces soft silken tofu

1 teaspoon pure vanilla extract

1 tablespoon melted vegan butter

oil for misting or cooking spray

1. Preheat the air fryer to 390°F.

2. In a medium bowl, combine the egg replacer and water and stir.

3. In a large bowl, stir together the flour, 2 tablespoons of sugar, baking powder, baking soda, and salt.

4. Add the tofu and vanilla to the egg mixture. Use a fork or whisk to break apart the tofu and blend until fairly smooth.

5. Stir in the melted vegan butter.

6. Add the tofu mixture to the dry ingredients and mix well. The dough may feel dry and crumbly. Use the back of a spoon to knead the dry crumbs into the mixture until you have a stiff dough that clings together.

7. Divide the dough into 16 portions and shape them into balls.

8. Mist the bites with oil and sprinkle the tops with the remaining coconut sugar.

9. Place 8 donut bites in the air fryer basket, leaving a little space around each. Cook for 4 to 5 minutes, until done in the center and lightly browned outside.

10. Repeat step 9 to cook the remaining donut bites.

English Muffin Breakfast Sandwich

Yield: 4 servings | Prep Time: 15 minutes | Cooking Time: 4–5 minutes per batch (2 batches) | Total Time: 23–25 minutes

KID FRIENDLY **SUPER EASY**

English muffins crisp up nicely in an air fryer and are so versatile. We love apples and vegan cheese, but you can use our method to experiment with your own favorite breakfast sandwich fillings.

1 medium red apple

4 whole English muffins

3/4 cup Cheddar-style shreds

ground cinnamon

1/4 cup coarsely chopped walnuts

1/4 cup dried cranberries

1. Preheat the air fryer to 390°F.

2. Quarter and core the apple and cut each quarter lengthwise into 1/4-inch slices.

3. Split 2 of the English muffins and lay them cut-side up.

4. On each bottom half, place a heaping tablespoon of cheese shreds and a quarter of the apple slices, which will overlap slightly. Sprinkle with cinnamon to taste.

5. On each top half, place 1 tablespoon of nuts and 1 tablespoon of cranberries. Top with a heaping tablespoon of cheese.

6. Place all 4 halves in the air fryer basket. They don't have to sit completely flat. To make all 4 fit, you may need to let them overlap a little.

7. Cook for 4 to 5 minutes or until the muffins heat through and are crispy on the bottom.

8. Transfer to a plate. Close each muffin and use a spatula to press the tops down firmly.

9. While the first batch is cooking, repeat above steps to assemble remaining muffins. Cook as above and serve hot.

See insert A2 for recipe photo.

VARIATIONS: Try these with sliced pears and substitute sliced almonds for the walnuts. Omit cheese and in steps 4 and 5, spread each muffin half with 2 teaspoons of date paste. Substitute chopped pecans or toasted sunflower seeds for the walnuts.

Flourless Oat Muffins

Yield: 8 muffins | Prep Time: 10 minutes | Cooking Time: 6–8 minutes per batch (2 batches) | Total Time: 22–26 minutes

GLUTEN FREE   TASTER FAVORITE

If you don't have any mashed sweet potatoes handy for this recipe, try canned pumpkin. Both will give you a substantial muffin that tastes like a chewy granola bar.

1¼ cups rolled oats

¼ cup oat bran

¼ teaspoon ground ginger

¼ teaspoon salt (optional)

¼ cup chopped pecans

½ cup mashed sweet potatoes

3 tablespoons molasses

8 silicone muffin cups

oil for misting or cooking spray

1. Preheat the air fryer to 360°F.

2. In a large bowl, stir together the oats, oat bran, ginger, salt, and pecans.

3. Add the sweet potatoes and molasses and stir until combined. The mixture will feel stiff, but make sure to distribute the sweet potatoes evenly.

4. Spray the muffin cups lightly with oil or cooking spray to prevent sticking.

5. Divide the mixture evenly among 8 muffin cups and pack them tightly. The cups will be full, but these muffins don't rise while baking.

6. Place 4 muffins in the air fryer basket and cook for 6 to 8 minutes. The tops should turn dark brown, but be careful not to let them burn.

7. Repeat step 6 to cook the remaining muffins.

> **NOTE:** We highly recommend silicone muffin cups for this recipe because they're easier to use when packing this stiff mixture. To use foil or paper cups, place them in a muffin tin while stuffing, then transfer to air fryer basket.
>
> **VARIATION:** Substitute ½ cup mashed canned pumpkin for the sweet potatoes.

Lemon-Blueberry Crepes

Yield: 4 servings | Prep Time: 10 minutes | Cooking Time: 4 minutes | Total Time: 14 minutes

FAST   GREAT SNACK   TASTER FAVORITE

No, they're not really crepes. Flour tortillas make these super quick and easy, and they taste great with this delightful, lemony filling.

1/4 cup soft silken tofu, drained (about 2 ounces)

3 tablespoons cream cheese

1 teaspoon grated lemon zest

1/2 teaspoon lemon juice

1 1/2 teaspoons coconut sugar

1/2 cup fresh blueberries

4 (8-inch) flour tortillas

1. Preheat the air fryer to 390°F.

2. In a food processor, combine the tofu, cream cheese, lemon zest, lemon juice, and sugar and process until smooth.

3. Place 1 tablespoon of filling on each tortilla and spread evenly to within 1/2-inch of the edges.

4. Top each tortilla with 2 tablespoons of blueberries, placing them in a line close to one edge. Roll up.

5. Place 2 tortillas in the air fryer basket. Place the other 2 on top, crosswise.

6. Cook for 4 minutes or just until the crepes heat through and brown lightly on the outside.

See insert A3 for recipe photo.

VARIATION: Omit lemon zest and juice. Add 1/8 teaspoon almond extract to filling (in step 2). Substitute 1/2 cup dried cherries for the blueberries.

Oatmeal Bars

Yield: varies | Prep Time: 5 minutes | Cooking Time: 7–9 minutes | Total Time: 12–14 minutes

FAST   GLUTEN FREE   SUPER EASY

Leftover oatmeal works great for this recipe if you follow step 1 so it won't be too thick. If starting with freshly cooked oatmeal, it will need to chill for at least 2 hours or overnight.

---

oatmeal

oil for misting or cooking spray

shredded coconut

finely chopped pecans

maple syrup for serving

1. Prepare the oatmeal according to the package directions.

2. While the oatmeal is still warm, pour it into a square or rectangular baking pan. It should be about ½-inch thick. If thicker than that, transfer some of it into another pan.

3. Chill several hours or overnight, until the oatmeal feels cold and firm.

4. When ready to cook, cut the oatmeal into 3-inch to 4-inch squares.

5. Cut each square in half to make rectangles or triangles.

6. Mist the bottoms of the oatmeal slices with oil or cooking spray.

7. Sprinkle the tops lightly with coconut and chopped pecans, pressing them in gently, then spray the tops with oil.

8. Place the slices in the air fryer basket in a single layer, close but not touching, and cook at 390°F for 7 to 9 minutes or until the tops turn brown and crispy.

9. Transfer the bars to serving plates. If any toppings fall off during cooking, sprinkle them over the bars and serve them hot with maple syrup.

NOTE: If you cook multiple batches, the second and subsequent batches will cook faster because the air fryer will be hot from cooking the previous batch(es).

TIP: These taste absolutely delicious with the Strawberry Jam (page 11).

Peanut Butter Breakfast Sticks

Yield: 4 servings | Prep Time: 10 minutes | Cooking Time: 4–6 minutes | Total Time: 14–16 minutes

FAST   GREAT SNACK   KID FRIENDLY   TASTER FAVORITE

Think of this recipe as a breakfast sundae. Bananas aren't your only option here. Try your own favorite sliced fruits or berries and add extra toppings such as chopped nuts or toasted coconut.

2 tablespoons Bob's Red Mill egg replacer

¼ cup water

½ cup crushed cornflake crumbs

day-old French bread or baguette loaf

6 tablespoons almond milk

1 teaspoon pure vanilla extract

½ teaspoon cinnamon

2 teaspoons coconut sugar

oil for misting or cooking spray

½ cup peanut butter

2 large bananas, sliced

1. In a shallow dish, mix together the egg replacer and water.

2. Place the cornflake crumbs in another shallow dish.

3. Preheat the air fryer to 390°F.

4. Cut the bread into "sticks" approximately 1 x 1 x 4 inches. Don't worry about being exact. Bread sticks will vary in size due to the shape of the loaf, and that's fine. Aim for 4 or 5 sticks per serving.

5. Add the almond milk, vanilla, cinnamon, and sugar to the egg mixture. Whisk together well.

6. Dip the bread sticks into the egg wash, shake off the excess, roll in the crumbs, then mist with oil or cooking spray.

7. Place the sticks in the air fryer basket in a single layer and cook for 3 to 4 minutes, until they turn brown and crispy. Transfer to serving plates.

8. Place the peanut butter in the air fryer baking pan and cook at 390°F for 1 minute. Stir and cook for 30 seconds to 1 minute longer, just until it warms.

9. Top each serving of breakfast sticks with sliced bananas and a generous drizzle of warm peanut butter.

> **NOTE:** You can stack the sticks in the basket as long as you place them crosswise to allow plenty of air flow around them.

Portabella Bacon

Yield: 2 servings | Prep Time: 15 minutes | Cooking Time: 7 minutes per batch (2 batches) | Total Time: 29 minutes

GLUTEN FREE **TASTER FAVORITE**

The flavor of these strips tastes amazingly like bacon. Our testers couldn't stop eating them! Try them on a sandwich with vegan mayonnaise and fresh tomatoes for a VLT.

2 large portabella mushrooms, stems removed

1 teaspoon smoked paprika

2 teaspoons maple syrup

1/8 teaspoon salt

2 tablespoons oil

1. Clean the portabellas and scrape out the gills with the tip of a knife.

2. Slice 1/4-inch thick and spread the slices on a cutting board.

3. In a small bowl, mix together the smoked paprika, maple syrup, salt, and oil.

4. Brush the seasoned oil on both sides of the mushroom slices.

5. Lay half the slices in the air fryer basket in a single layer.

6. Cook at 390°F for 7 minutes, until they brown. They won't be crispy.

7. Repeat steps 5 and 6 to cook the remaining strips.

> **TIP:** Soaking mushrooms in water to clean them will give you soggy or spongy mushrooms. The best way to clean them is with a clean damp cloth or vegetable brush.

Strawberry Jam

Yield: 1 cup | Prep Time: 10 minutes | Cooking Time: 15 minutes | Total Time: 25 minutes

GLUTEN FREE   KID FRIENDLY   SUPER EASY

This recipe tastes tart yet sweet. The fresh flavor of the strawberries shines through like morning sun through a kitchen window.

1 pound fresh strawberries, coarsely chopped

½ teaspoon grated lemon peel

1 teaspoon lemon juice

1 cup sugar

1. In a food processor or blender, puree the strawberries.

2. Pour them into a mixing bowl, add the lemon peel, juice, and sugar, and mix together.

3. Pour the strawberry mixture into the air fryer baking pan.

4. Cook at 390°F for 5 minutes.

5. Stir and cook for 5 more minutes.

6. Stir again and cook for 5 additional minutes.

7. Pour into a bowl and cool to room temperature.

NOTE: Use freshly squeezed lemon juice for this recipe—no bright yellow squeeze bottles of flavored water!

Also, this recipe creates a soft jam that will thicken in the fridge, which is where you should store it. Jam will keep for 2 to 3 weeks.

VARIATION: Use raspberries or blueberries (or a mixture) in place of strawberries.

Sweet Potato Toast

Yield: 6–8 slices | Prep Time: 5 minutes | Cooking Time: 6 minutes | Total Time: 11 minutes

FAST   GLUTEN FREE   GREAT SNACK   SUPER EASY

This recipe is super versatile, and the possibilities are endless. We use date paste for a sweet version, but you can make your own toast base and get creative with the toppings. Cooking it in your air fryer also makes it faster and less messy.

1 small sweet potato

oil for misting

Date Paste (page 152)

1–2 tablespoons grated coconut

sliced almonds and dried cranberries for topping

1. Preheat the air fryer to 390°F.

2. Cut the sweet potato into slices between $\frac{1}{4}$-inch and $\frac{1}{2}$-inch thick.

3. Spray one side of the sweet potato slices with oil.

4. Flip them over and spread a layer of Date Paste to taste on the other side.

5. Sprinkle the coconut lightly onto the Date Paste, pressing to make it stick.

6. Place the potato slices in the air fryer basket in a single layer.

7. Cook for about 6 minutes until the potato slices are barely fork tender.

8. Before serving, top the sweet potatoes with sliced almonds and dried cranberries, or sprinkle them with the spices or toppings of your choice.

VARIATION: For savory sweet potato toast, omit the date paste.

Taquitos & Jam

Yield: 8 taquitos | Prep Time: 12 minutes | Cooking Time: 4–5 minutes per batch (2 batches) | Total Time: 20–22 minutes

GLUTEN FREE

With peanut butter as your base, almost anything goes with this crispy breakfast treat. Check out the variations below.

½ cup peanut butter

½ cup coconut chips or ½ cup shredded coconut

2 tablespoons sunflower seeds

8 (8-inch) corn tortillas

oil for misting or cooking spray

Strawberry Jam (page 11) for dipping

1. Preheat the air fryer to 390°F.

2. In a medium bowl, mix together the peanut butter, coconut, and sunflower seeds.

3. To soften the tortillas, wrap them in damp paper towels and microwave them on high for 45 to 60 seconds, until they're warm.

4. Prepare the tortillas one at a time, keeping the others covered with the steamy paper towels.

5. Spray one side with oil or cooking spray.

6. Flip it over and place a rounded tablespoon of peanut butter filling on the other side, spreading it evenly to cover about half of the tortilla.

7. Roll up the tortilla loosely and lay it seam side down while you prepare 3 more.

8. Place 4 taquitos in the air fryer basket in a single layer. Cook for 4 to 5 minutes, until they lightly brown.

9. Repeat steps 5 through 8 to fill and cook the remaining taquitos.

10. The filling will be very hot, so allow the taquitos to cool slightly, then serve them warm with the strawberry jam for dipping.

NOTE: Whatever fillings you choose, be careful not to overfill the taquitos. Have fun experimenting with your own favorite combinations.

VARIATIONS: For the sunflower seeds, substitute pumpkin seeds, finely chopped walnuts, or pecans. Instead of coconut, try raisins, dried cranberries, or chopped dates.

Toast, Plain & Simple

Yield: 2 pieces | Prep Time: 1 minute | Cooking Time: 3–5 minutes | Total Time: 4–5 minutes

FAST   GREAT SNACK   SUPER EASY

Air fryers have become the go-to appliance in our kitchens. A toaster does just one thing—so why use it anymore? See the Tip below for the best toasting breads.

2 slices bread

1. Cut bread slices in half for a better fit.
2. Place the slices in the air fryer basket and cook at 360°F for 3 minutes.
3. Flip them over and cook 1 to 2 minutes longer until they brown on both sides.

> **TIP:** Ordinary wheat and white sandwich bread slices work well, as does commercial oat-nut bread. Heavily seeded and sprouted grain breads, however, may tend to cook unevenly.

Veggie Sausage Corn Muffins

Yield: 10 muffins | Prep Time: 12 minutes | Cooking Time: crumbles 5–6 minutes; muffins 10–12 minutes per batch (2 batches) | Total Time: 37–42 minutes

TASTER FAVORITE

You can use foil muffin cups, but we strongly recommend using oven-safe silicone cups. Using plain meatless crumbles gives you total control over taste. Love sage? Add more. Hate sage? Omit it altogether or replace it with your favorite herb or spice.

Veggie Sausage

oil for misting or cooking spray

1 cup veggie ground crumbles

1/4 teaspoon dried thyme

1/4 teaspoon rubbed sage

1/8 teaspoon ground allspice

1/8 teaspoon ground nutmeg

Corn Muffins

1 tablespoon flaxseed meal

2 tablespoons water

10 silicone muffin cups

3/4 cup all-purpose white flour

3/4 cup yellow cornmeal

2 1/2 teaspoons baking powder

1/4 teaspoon salt

3/4 cup almond milk

3 tablespoons vegan butter, melted

applesauce (optional)

Strawberry Jam (page 11) for serving (optional)

> **VARIATION:** Instead of using ground crumbles, you can substitute 1 cup of cooked, crumbled, meatless breakfast sausage.

1. Spray the air fryer baking pan lightly with oil or cooking spray, add all veggie sausage ingredients, and stir.

2. Cook at 390°F for 5 to 6 minutes, stirring at 2-minute intervals, until done. Set aside.

3. Meanwhile, in a medium bowl, stir together the flaxseed meal and water and set aside.

4. If using foil muffin cups, remove the paper liners and save for another use. Again, we recommend silicone.

5. Spray the muffin cups lightly with oil or cooking spray.

6. Preheat the air fryer to 390°F.

7. In a large bowl, stir together the flour, cornmeal, baking powder, and salt.

8. Add the milk and melted butter to the flaxseed mixture and whisk it together.

9. Pour the flaxseed mixture into the dry ingredients and mix well.

10. Stir in the cooked veggie sausage crumbles.

11. Spoon the mixture into the prepared muffin cups.

12. Place 5 muffin cups in the air fryer basket and cook for 10 to 12 minutes or until a toothpick inserted into the center comes out clean.

13. Repeat step 11 and 12 to bake the remaining muffins.

14. To serve, split open the muffins and top them with warm applesauce or Strawberry Jam (page 11).

APPETIZERS & SNACKS

Artichoke Balls

Yield: 15 balls | Prep Time: 26 minutes | Cooking Time: 10 minutes | Total Time: 36 minutes

GREAT SNACK   SUPER EASY   TASTER FAVORITE

These balls offer a new take on an old cocktail-party standby.

---

1 (14-ounce) can artichoke hearts, drained

1 cup panko breadcrumbs

1 tablespoon extra-virgin olive oil

1 teaspoon vegan Worcestershire sauce

2 tablespoons grated Parmesan-style topping

1 cup nut milk of choice

1 tablespoon thinly sliced green onions

1. Using your hands, smash all ingredients together to make a stiff mixture.

2. Shape 1 tablespoon at a time into a smooth, cohesive ball.

3. Place the artichoke balls in the air fryer, close together but not touching.

4. Cook at 390°F for 10 minutes. Serve warm or at room temperature.

TIP: We recommend wearing kitchen gloves when handling messy mixtures with the hands.

Asparagus Fries

Yield: 4 servings | Prep Time: 15 minutes | Cooking Time: 5–7 minutes per batch (2 batches) | Total Time: 25–29 minutes

GREAT SNACK TASTER FAVORITE

Lemon and parmesan add lively flavor to these fabulous fries, and your air fryer lets you indulge without the guilt of deep frying.

---

2 tablespoons Bob's Red Mill egg replacer

4 tablespoons water

3/4 cup panko breadcrumbs

1/4 cup grated Parmesan-style topping

1/4 teaspoon salt

1 teaspoon lemon pepper seasoning

12 ounces fresh asparagus spears, tough ends removed

3 tablespoons almond milk

oil for misting or cooking spray

1. Preheat the air fryer to 390°F.

2. In a small bowl, stir together the egg replacer and water. Set aside to thicken.

3. Place the breadcrumbs, Parmesan topping, salt, and lemon pepper in a sealable plastic bag or container with a lid. Shake to mix well.

4. If the asparagus spears are longer than the width of your air fryer basket, snap them in half. Place the spears in another sealable plastic bag or container with lid.

5. Add the milk to the egg mixture and whisk to combine.

6. Pour the milk mixture over the asparagus. Seal the bag or close the lid and shake to coat thoroughly.

7. Remove the spears from the egg wash, letting the excess drip off.

8. Place the spears in the bag or container with the panko mixture and shake until they coat evenly.

9. Place a single layer of asparagus spears in the air fryer basket, leaving a little space around each of them. Mist the spears with oil or cooking spray.

10. Stack another layer on top crosswise and mist. Continue until you've used about half the asparagus but no more than 4 or 5 layers.

11. Cook for 5 to 7 minutes, until they turn crispy and golden brown. If needed, shake and mist again during cooking to coat any spots that aren't browning.

12. Repeat steps 9 through 11 to cook the remaining spears.

TIP: Save the woody ends of the asparagus for making your next batch of veggie broth.

Avocado Fries

Yield: 4 servings | Prep Time: 5 minutes | Cooking Time: 10 minutes | Total Time: 15 minutes

FAST   GREAT SNACK   TASTER FAVORITE

Deep-fried avocados aren't healthy—but they taste so delicious. This recipe allows you to enjoy a rich treat with less guilt.

1/4 cup almond milk or coconut milk

1 tablespoon lime juice

1/8 teaspoon Tabasco sauce

3/4 cup panko breadcrumbs

1/4 cup cornmeal

1/4 teaspoon salt

2 tablespoons flour

1 large avocado

oil for misting or cooking spray

1. In a small bowl, whisk together the milk, lime juice, and Tabasco sauce.

2. In a shallow dish, mix together the panko, cornmeal, and salt.

3. In another shallow dish, place the flour.

4. Halve the avocado and remove the pit.

5. Use a spoon to lift the avocado halves from the skin.

6. Cut each avocado half crosswise into 1/2-inch slices.

7. Dip the slices in flour, then the milk mixture, and then roll them in the breadcrumbs.

8. Mist with oil or cooking spray.

9. Cook at 390°F for 10 minutes, until the coating becomes brown and crispy. Serve warm.

Avocado Taquitos

Yield: 4 servings | Prep Time: 15 minutes | Cooking Time: 6–8 minutes per batch (2 batches) | Total Time: 27–31 minutes

GLUTEN FREE GREAT SNACK

Pile on the jalapeño slices and Sriracha sauce to make these as hot as you like. To cool down, consider an ice-cold fruit smoothie for dessert.

Filling
1/2 cup refried pinto beans
1/2 cup Monterey Jack & Cheddar–style shreds
1/4 cup corn kernels
2 tablespoons chopped green onion (tops)
1/2 teaspoon lime juice
1/2 teaspoon garlic powder
1/2 teaspoon chili powder
1/2 teaspoon cumin

1 medium avocado
12 (6- to 7-inch) corn tortillas
oil for misting or cooking spray
chili powder for coating
salsa or Sriracha sauce (optional)

1. Mix together all filling ingredients and set aside.
2. Halve the avocado and remove the pit.
3. Use a spoon to lift the avocado halves from the skin.
4. Cut the avocado lengthwise into 12 thin slices.
5. Warm the tortillas for easier rolling by wrapping them in damp paper towels and microwaving them on high for 30 to 60 seconds.
6. One at a time, place 1 tablespoon of filling on each tortilla. Top with a sliver of avocado and roll up. Secure with toothpicks.
7. Spray the taquito with oil or cooking spray and sprinkle with chili powder.
8. Place 6 taquitos in the air fryer basket, 4 on the bottom layer and 2 stacked crosswise on top. Cook at 390°F for 6 to 8 minutes, until they turn crispy and brown.
9. Repeat step 8 to cook remaining taquitos.
10. Serve plain or with salsa or Sriracha sauce for dipping.

TIP: If using frozen corn for this recipe, measure *after* thawing and draining.

Banana Fries

Yield: 4–6 servings | Prep Time: 10 minutes | Cooking Time: 4–5 minutes per batch (2 batches) | Total Time: 18–20 minutes

GREAT SNACK KID FRIENDLY

Ripe bananas fall apart in the coating process and then cook to mush, so use only very firm bananas for this recipe. If they're still almost green at the stem end, they will hold up well for coating and soften perfectly when cooked.

½ cup crushed cornflakes

½ cup finely chopped peanuts

¼ cup potato starch

¼ cup maple syrup

2 firm bananas

oil for misting or cooking spray

1. Preheat the air fryer to 390°F.

2. In a shallow dish, mix together the cornflake crumbs and peanuts.

3. In another shallow dish, place the potato starch.

4. Into a third shallow dish, pour the syrup.

5. Cut the bananas in half crosswise. Cut each half in quarters lengthwise so that you have 16 "sticks."

6. Dip the banana sticks in potato starch and tap to shake off excess.

7. Dip the bananas in the syrup, roll in the crumb mixture, and spray with oil or cooking spray.

8. Place the banana sticks in the air fryer basket in a single layer. If need be, you can stack a few crosswise, but don't overcrowd the basket or they won't brown well.

9. Cook for 4 to 5 minutes or until golden brown and crispy.

10. Repeat steps 8 and 9 to cook the remaining bananas.

Battered Cauliflower

Yield: 3–4 servings | Prep Time: 27 minutes | Cooking Time: 15 minutes | Total Time: 42 minutes

GREAT SNACK

Fried cauliflower tastes delicious as is, but for a tasty treat try enjoying it with Curry Dip (page 31).

Batter

1 cup all-purpose white flour

1 tablespoon ground flaxseed

1⅓ cups almond milk

2 cups panko breadcrumbs

Cauliflower

2 teaspoons dried tarragon

1 teaspoon parsley

1 tablespoon unbleached flour

½ teaspoon salt

1 (12-ounce) package frozen cauliflower florets, thawed and drained

oil for misting

1. In a medium bowl, mix all the batter ingredients together and set aside.

2. On a sheet of wax paper, pour the breadcrumbs.

3. In a small bowl, mix the tarragon, parsley, flour, and salt together.

4. Stir the seasoning mixture into the cauliflower to coat the florets evenly.

5. Dip the cauliflower florets in the batter and roll in the breadcrumbs.

6. Mist all sides with oil and cook at 390°F for 10 minutes

7. Flip the florets and cook for an additional 5 minutes, until they become brown and crisp.

See insert A4 for recipe photo.

Bell Pepper Rings

Yield: 4 servings | Prep Time: 15 minutes | Cooking Time: 13–14 minutes | Total Time: 28–29 minutes

GREAT SNACK   TASTER FAVORITE

Some people think these tasty snacks are an ugly-duckling substitute for onion rings, but what they lack in looks they make up for in fabulous flavor.

2 large bell peppers

½ cup all-purpose white flour

½ teaspoon salt

½ cup lemon-lime soda

½ cup crushed panko breadcrumbs

½ cup plain breadcrumbs

oil for misting or cooking spray

1. Preheat the air fryer to 390°F.

2. Slice the bell peppers widthwise into ¼-inch rings. Remove the seeds and membranes.

3. In a large bowl, stir together the flour and salt.

4. Slowly pour the soda into the flour mixture and stir until the foaming stops and you have a medium-thick batter.

5. Place the pepper rings in the batter and stir until thoroughly coated.

6. Place panko and plain breadcrumbs in a plastic bag or a container with a lid. Shake to mix.

7. Working with a few at a time, remove the pepper rings from the batter and shake off the excess.

8. Place the battered rings in the breadcrumb bag or container. Shake to coat the rings, then lay them on a baking sheet or wax paper.

9. After breading all the rings, spray them with oil and transfer them to the air fryer basket. The rings can overlap in layers but arrange them with plenty of gaps to allow for air circulation while cooking.

10. Cook for 10 minutes. Use tongs or a fork to rearrange rings and mist any white spots with oil.

11. Cook for an additional 3 to 4 minutes, until golden brown and crispy.

NOTE: You can use full-sugar or diet soda for this recipe.

TIP: For bright, vivid color, we suggest using 1 red bell pepper and 1 yellow bell pepper—but green works just fine too.

Cauliflower Spring Rolls with Peanut Sauce

Yield: 8 spring rolls | Prep Time: 20 minutes | Cooking Time: 20 minutes per batch (2 batches) | Total Time: 1 hour

GLUTEN FREE   GREAT SNACK

In the mood for something a little different than the usual spring roll? This one with its spicy sauce will do the trick. It's sure to impress as an appetizer at your next dinner party.

---

1 (12-ounce) bag riced cauliflower, thawed

¼ cup dried currants

¼ cup coconut milk

1 teaspoon curry powder

½ teaspoon cinnamon

2 tablespoons minced green onions

¼ teaspoon salt

8 (8-inch) rice paper wrappers

oil for misting or cooking spray

Peanut Sauce

½ cup creamy peanut butter

1 tablespoon maple syrup

1 tablespoon lemon or lime juice

½ teaspoon garlic powder

1 tablespoon minced onion

¼ teaspoon crushed red pepper flakes

1. In a large bowl, mix together the cauliflower rice, currants, coconut milk, curry powder, cinnamon, green onions, and salt.

2. Divide the filling into 8 equal portions.

3. Quickly dip 1 rice paper wrapper in lukewarm (approximately 105°F) water to soften.

4. Spoon 1 portion of the filling down the center of the rice paper wrapper.

5. Fold 2 sides in and then roll it up like a burrito. Set aside on wax paper.

6. Repeat steps 3 through 5 with 3 more sheets of rice paper.

7. Mist all sides of the spring rolls with oil or cooking spray and place 4 in the air fryer basket.

8. Cook at 390°F for 10 minutes. Turn and cook 10 more minutes, until brown and crispy.

9. Repeat steps 3 through 8 for the second batch of spring rolls.

10. While the spring rolls are cooking, make the Peanut Sauce by processing all sauce ingredients in a food processor or blender until smooth.

VARIATION: Substitute raisins, dried cherries, or dried cranberries for the currants.

Cereal Snack Mix

Yield: 8 (½ cup) servings | Prep Time: 5 minutes | Cooking Time: 7 minutes | Total Time: 12 minutes

FAST   GREAT SNACK   KID FRIENDLY   SUPER EASY

This recipe is great for a road trip or hike, and kids love it too.

4 cups crispy rice cereal

¼ teaspoon salt

2 teaspoons dill

3 tablespoons grated Parmesan-style topping

1 tablespoon soy sauce

1. In a medium bowl, stir all ingredients together to coat well.

2. Pour into the air fryer baking pan.

3. Cook at 360°F for 5 minutes.

4. Stir and cook for 2 more minutes.

VARIATION: After you've made this a few times, play around with the ingredients. Substitute your favorite herbs and spices—but always include 1 tablespoon of liquid (soy sauce, olive oil, vegan teriyaki sauce, hot pepper sauce, maple syrup) so the dry ingredients can stick to the cereal. You also can use different types of dry cereal, small pretzels, or even peanuts. However you mix and match, keep the ratio at 1 tablespoon liquid to 4 cups dry.

Cheddar-Olive Nuggets

Yield: 24–26 nuggets | Prep Time: 20 minutes | Cooking Time: 13–15 minutes per batch (2 batches) | Total Time: 46–50 minutes

GREAT SNACK

For a delicious blend of salty and sweet, try dipping these little nuggets in Strawberry Jam. Olives not your thing? Try the tea biscuit variation below, which also tastes delicious dipped in the Strawberry Jam.

---

1 (7-ounce) jar pimento-stuffed green olives

1 cup Monterey Jack & Cheddar–style shreds

1 cup self-rising flour

$1\frac{1}{2}$ tablespoons all-vegetable shortening

3 tablespoons almond milk

oil for misting

Strawberry Jam (page 11) (optional)

1. Drain the olives and blot them dry on paper towels.
2. Chop the cheese shreds and place them in a medium bowl.
3. Add the flour to the cheese shreds and mix together with your hands.
4. Still using your hands, work the shortening into the mixture until it's well blended.
5. Work in the milk until a dough forms.
6. Using $1\frac{1}{2}$ teaspoons of dough for each olive, roll the dough into a ball, then flatten the ball into a disc about $2\frac{1}{2}$ inches in diameter.
7. Lay the olive in the center of the dough and wrap the dough around the olive, squeezing and pinching to seal it.
8. Repeat to make 12 or 13 nuggets.
9. Mist the nuggets with oil and place them in the air fryer basket in a single layer.
10. Cook at 390°F for 13 to 15 minutes, until they brown.
11. Repeat steps 6 through 10 to cook the remaining nuggets.
12. Serve with Strawberry Jam for dipping if you like.

NOTE: Reserve the olive brine to store any unused olives . . . or use it to make a dirty martini for sipping while the nuggets cook!

TIP: This dough will want to stick to your fingers when you're mixing and shaping it. Food-grade gloves will make for less mess.

VARIATION: Cheddar Tea Biscuits: Omit the olives and prepare steps 2 through 5 as above. Using the same amount of dough, shape into a ball and flatten to 1½-inch diameter. Mist both sides and place in the basket in a single layer. Cook at 390°F for 8 to 10 minutes, until brown. You'll need to cook these in 2 batches as well.

Chickenless Crispy Sandwich

Yield: 1 serving | Prep Time: 5 minutes | Cooking Time: 20 minutes | Total Time: 25 minutes

GREAT SNACK **SUPER EASY**

Try this sandwich for a quick and tasty lunch.

---

1 breaded chicken-style patty

1 tablespoon vegan mayonnaise

½ teaspoon poultry seasoning

1 sandwich bun

1 leaf lettuce

1 slice tomato

Pickled Red Onions (page 155)

1. Cook the patty in the basket of the air fryer at 390°F for 10 minutes.

2. Flip it over and cook for an additional 10 minutes.

3. Meanwhile, in a small bowl, stir the vegan mayonnaise and poultry seasoning together.

4. Spread the seasoned mayonnaise on both pieces of the bun.

5. Place the cooked patty on the bottom half of the bun.

6. Add the lettuce, tomato, and Pickled Red Onions and top with the upper half of the bun.

NOTE: We recommend Gardein Crispy Chick'n Patty for this recipe.

VARIATION: Substitute Pecan-Crusted Eggplant (page 67) for the chicken-style patty

Chickpeas for Snacking

Yield: approximately 1 cup | Prep Time: 5 minutes | Cooking Time: 12–15 minutes | Total Time: 17–20 minutes

GLUTEN FREE   GREAT SNACK   SUPER EASY

For best results, make sure your chickpeas are well drained and as dry as possible. Removing as much moisture as you can makes them crispier, which improves their taste and gives them a nice, satisfying crunch. Tex-Mex seasoning is our favorite, but check out the variations and try your own favorite combination of spices.

1 (15-ounce) can chickpeas, drained

2 teaspoons Tex-Mex Seasoning (page 159)

1/4 teaspoon salt

1 tablespoon olive oil

1. Drain the chickpeas and spread them in a single layer on a couple of paper towels.

2. Cover with another paper towel. Press gently and roll to remove extra moisture. Don't press too hard or you'll crush the chickpeas.

3. Place chickpeas in a medium bowl and sprinkle with seasoning. Stir to coat well.

4. Add the oil and stir again to distribute evenly.

5. Cook at 390°F for 12 to 15 minutes, shaking the basket about halfway through the cooking time.

6. Cool completely and store in an airtight container.

VARIATIONS:

SMOKEY HOT SEASONING

1/2 teaspoon smoked paprika

1/4 teaspoon onion powder

1/4 teaspoon garlic powder

1/8 teaspoon salt

cayenne pepper

FIVE SPICE

2 teaspoons Chinese Five-Spice powder

1/4 teaspoon salt

1 tablespoon sesame oil (instead of olive oil)

Chickpea-Sweet Potato Croquettes

Yield: 12 croquettes | Prep Time: 10 minutes | Cooking Time: 9 minutes | Total Time: 19 minutes

GREAT SNACK

The flavor of these tasty croquettes will remind you of falafels, but they're much faster and easier to make.

1 (15½-ounce) can chickpeas, drained

1 teaspoon ground cumin

½ teaspoon ground coriander seed

½ teaspoon garlic powder

½ teaspoon onion powder

½ cup mashed sweet potatoes

salt and pepper

½ cup crushed panko breadcrumbs

2 tablespoons sesame seeds

oil for misting or cooking spray

1. Preheat the air fryer to 390°F.

2. In a food processor, place half of the drained chickpeas and add the cumin, coriander, garlic, and onion powder. Process until the mixture becomes almost completely smooth. Transfer to a large bowl.

3. Process the remaining chickpeas with a few short pulses, just enough to rough chop them. Don't overdo it—some large chunks should remain.

4. Add the chopped chickpeas to the bowl with the smooth chickpeas. Add the sweet potatoes, salt and pepper to taste, and mix well.

5. Divide the mixture into 12 portions and shape into croquettes about 2 inches long. Press them tightly to make sure they hold together.

6. In a shallow dish, mix the breadcrumbs and sesame seeds.

7. Roll the croquettes in the crumb mixture, pressing them to make the coating stick.

8. Mist the croquettes with oil, place them in the air fryer basket in a single layer—close but not touching—and cook for 7 minutes.

9. Mist any light spots that aren't browning and cook for 2 more minutes or until golden brown.

Eggplant Fries with Curry Dip

Yield: 4 servings | Prep Time: 10 minutes | Cooking Time: 7–8 minutes per batch (2 batches) | Total Time: 24–26 minutes

GREAT SNACK   TASTER FAVORITE

You can save some calories in this dip by substituting mashed avocado for $1/4$ cup of the vegan mayo. We used the Follow Your Heart brand, but any good mayo will have enough acid to prevent the avocado from turning brown.

Curry Dip

$3/4$ cup vegan mayonnaise

$1^1/2$ teaspoons curry powder

$1/4$ teaspoon dry mustard

black pepper

hot sauce

Eggplant Fries

2 tablespoons Bob's Red Mill egg replacer

4 tablespoons water

1 medium eggplant

salt

1 cup crushed panko breadcrumbs

3 ounces almond milk

oil for misting or cooking spray

1. In a small bowl, combine all the dip ingredients and blend well. Cover and refrigerate while preparing fries.

2. In a large bowl, combine the egg replacer and water and set aside.

3. Peel and cut the eggplant into fat fries, roughly $3/8$- to $1/2$-inch thick. Retain the peel if you like the taste.

4. Preheat the air fryer to 390°F.

5. Sprinkle the eggplant fries with salt to taste.

6. Place the panko crumbs in a shallow dish.

7. Add the milk to the egg mixture and whisk to mix together well.

8. Add the eggplant fries to the egg wash and stir to coat.

9. Remove the fries from the egg wash, shaking off the excess, and roll them in the breadcrumbs.

10. Spray the fries on all sides with oil.

11. Place half of the fries in the air fryer basket in a single layer. It's fine if the fries crowd and overlap a little.

12. Cook for 5 minutes.

13. Shake the basket, lightly mist the fries with oil again, and cook for 2 to 3 minutes longer, until brown and crispy.

14. Repeat steps 11 through 13 to cook remaining fries.

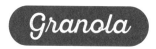

Granola

Yield: 2 cups | Prep Time: 10 minutes | Cooking Time: 7–10 minutes | Total Time: 17–20 minutes

GLUTEN FREE   GREAT SNACK

Granola is great for snacking and makes a tasty topping for fresh sliced fruits, warm or cold. If you're feeling adventurous, try substituting various nuts, seeds, and dried fruits in this recipe to create other flavorful combinations.

1 cup rolled oats

¼ cup shredded, unsweetened coconut

½ cup coarsely chopped walnuts

¼ cup pumpkin seeds

2 tablespoons sunflower seeds

1 tablespoon flaxseed meal

½ cup dried cranberries

¼ cup Date Paste (page 152)

2 tablespoons pure maple syrup

1 teaspoon vanilla extract

oil for misting or cooking spray

1. In a large bowl, stir together all dry ingredients.

2. In a small bowl, combine the Date Paste, syrup, and vanilla and stir until well blended.

3. Pour the syrup mixture over the dry ingredients. Stir until the dry ingredients are well coated.

4. Lightly spray the air fryer baking pan with oil or cooking spray.

5. Pour the granola into the pan and cook at 390°F for 5 minutes.

6. Stir and continue cooking for 2 to 5 minutes, stirring every minute or two, until golden brown. Watch closely—once the mixture begins to brown, it will cook quickly!

7. Remove the granola from the pan and spread on wax paper to cool.

8. Let the granola cool completely and store it in an airtight container.

See insert A5 for recipe photo.

Jalapeño Poppers

Yield: 18–20 | Prep Time: 1 hour | Cooking Time: 7–9 minutes | Total Time: 1 hour 7–9 minutes

GREAT SNACK

We prefer this somewhat mild version of this popular appetizer, but it's easy enough to add heat to taste: Instead of discarding the pepper seeds and membranes, chop some or all of them and stir into the filling.

Filling

4 ounces vegan cream cheese

1 teaspoon grated lime zest

$\frac{1}{4}$ teaspoon chili powder

$\frac{1}{8}$ teaspoon garlic powder

$\frac{1}{4}$ teaspoon salt

$\frac{1}{2}$ pound jalapeño peppers

1 tablespoon Bob's Red Mill egg replacer

1 tablespoon lime juice

3 tablespoons water

$\frac{1}{4}$ cup cornstarch

$\frac{1}{2}$ cup panko breadcrumbs

$\frac{1}{2}$ teaspoon salt

oil for misting or cooking spray

1. In a small bowl, mix together all the filling ingredients. Cover and refrigerate while preparing the peppers.

2. Cut the jalapeños into $\frac{1}{2}$-inch slices.

3. Using a sharp knife, remove the seeds and veins and discard, reserve for alternate use, or chop and mix into the filling for extra-hot poppers.

4. Stuff each pepper ring with filling.

5. In a shallow dish, combine the egg replacer, lime juice, and water.

6. In another shallow dish, place the cornstarch.

7. In a third shallow dish, stir together the breadcrumbs and salt.

8. Dip each pepper slice in cornstarch, shake off the excess, then dip in the egg mixture.

9. Roll the pepper slice in the breadcrumbs, pressing to make the coating stick.

10. Place the pepper slices on a plate in a single layer and freeze them for 30 minutes.

11. Preheat the air fryer to 390°F.

12. Spray the frozen peppers with oil or cooking spray, place them in the air fryer basket in a single layer, and cook for 5 minutes.

13. Mist any that aren't browning and cook for an additional 2 to 4 minutes or until the coating becomes browned and crispy.

NOTE: The size of the rings will vary, so these may cook unevenly. If that happens, use tongs to remove the poppers that have finished cooking while the others cook longer.

Jalapeño-Tofu Sliders

Yield: 16 sliders | Prep Time: 15 minutes | Cooking Time: 6–7 minutes per batch (2 batches) | Total Time: 27–29 minutes

GREAT SNACK

Fresh is always best, but sometimes speed and convenience are important too. Keep a jar of jalapeños in the pantry, and you can throw together all sorts of treats in just a few minutes.

---

1 (14-ounce) package firm silken tofu

½ cup bottled jalapeño slices, drained and roughly chopped

½ teaspoon salt

½ teaspoon onion powder

2 tablespoons Frank's hot sauce

2 cups panko breadcrumbs, divided

3–4 tablespoons potato starch

oil for misting or cooking spray

Spread

½ cup vegan sour cream

½ cup vegan mayonnaise

3 tablespoons coarse brown mustard

2 teaspoons Frank's hot sauce

16 slider buns

3–4 small tomatoes, thinly sliced

lettuce

1. Preheat the air fryer to 390°F.

2. Drain the tofu, pat it dry, and grate it into a large bowl.

3. Add the jalapeños, salt, onion powder, hot sauce, and 1½ cups panko and mix well.

4. If needed, stir in the potato starch to help bind the mixture together. It should feel moist yet firm enough to hold its shape when formed into patties.

5. In a shallow dish, place the remaining ½ cup of panko.

6. Shape the tofu mixture into 16 slider-size patties.

7. Roll the patties gently in panko, pressing slightly to make the coating stick.

8. Mist the patties with oil, place 8 of them in the air fryer basket, and cook for 6 to 7 minutes, until golden brown.

9. Repeat to cook the remaining patties.

10. Meanwhile, in a small bowl, combine all of the spread ingredients and mix thoroughly.

11. To serve, place the patties on warmed slider buns and top with tomatoes, lettuce, and spread.

Mini Tacos

Yield: 24 mini tacos | Prep Time: 10 minutes | Cooking Time: 8–10 minutes per batch (2 batches) | Total Time: 26–30 minutes

GLUTEN FREE   GREAT SNACK   SUPER EASY

Often called street tacos, these small snacks are meant for easy eating on the go. They're also great for a sit-down meal where you can pile on extra jalapeños and Sriracha for all the heat you want.

24 (4-inch) corn tortillas

1½ cups refried beans (about ¾ of a 15-ounce can)

1 small jar jalapeño slices

1 cup Monterey Jack–style shreds

½ cup salsa

oil for misting or cooking spray

Sriracha sauce (optional)

1. Preheat the air fryer to 390°F.

2. To soften the tortillas, wrap them in damp paper towels and microwave them on high for 30 to 60 seconds.

3. One tortilla at a time, top with 1 tablespoon of beans, 1 or 2 jalapeño slices, 1 tablespoon of vegan cheese, and 1 teaspoon of salsa.

4. Fold the tortilla over, press down gently on the center, then press the edges firmly all around to seal. Spray both sides with oil or cooking spray.

5. Place half of the tacos in the air fryer basket. To fit 12 in the basket, you can stand them upright and lean some against the sides. Crowding is OK as long as you leave a little room for air circulation.

6. Cook for 8 to 10 minutes or until golden brown and crispy.

7. Repeat steps 5 and 6 to cook the remaining tacos.

8. Serve as is or top with Sriracha sauce and more jalapeños.

> **TIP:** You can rewarm the tortillas as needed to keep them soft enough to fold without breaking.

Pickled Okra Fries

Yield: 2–4 servings | Prep Time: 10 minutes | Cooking Time: 11–12 minutes | Total Time: 21–22 minutes

GREAT SNACK   KID FRIENDLY   TASTER FAVORITE

Strange as it may seem, this is a kid favorite at our houses. If you like fried pickles, then you really must try fried pickled okra!

1 tablespoon Bob's Red Mill egg replacer

2 tablespoons water

1 (16-ounce) jar pickled okra

½ cup panko breadcrumbs

½ cup masa harina flour

3 tablespoons almond milk

oil for misting or cooking spray

1. In a bowl large enough to hold all the okra, mix together the egg replacer and water. Set aside to thicken.

2. Drain the okra and cut each pod in half lengthwise.

3. Place the panko and masa harina in a large plastic bag or container with lid. Shake or stir to mix together well.

4. Preheat the air fryer to 390°F.

5. Whisk the almond milk into the egg mixture until smooth.

6. Add the okra to the egg wash and stir gently to coat.

7. Remove the okra from the egg wash, letting the excess drip off. Place the okra slices in the panko mixture and shake to coat.

8. Pile the breaded okra in the air fryer basket and spray with oil or cooking spray.

9. Cook for 5 minutes.

10. Shake the basket to rearrange the pieces, spray with more oil or cooking spray, and cook for 5 more minutes.

11. Shake to separate any okra pieces that are sticking together. Spray again to coat any spots you've missed. Cook for 1 to 2 minutes longer or until lightly brown and crispy.

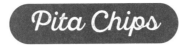

Pita Chips

Yield: 4 servings | Prep Time: 5 minutes | Cooking Time: 4–6 minutes | Total Time: 9–11 minutes

FAST   GREAT SNACK   SUPER EASY

Satisfy your craving for a crunchy snack with these tasty chips. They have plenty of flavor on their own, but they also go well with soups, salads, hummus, and dips. Our favorite is the Texas Two-Step Dip (page 160).

2 (6-inch) pitas

1¼ teaspoons Tex-Mex Seasoning (page 159)

¼ teaspoon salt

oil for misting or cooking spray

1. Cut each pita half into 4 wedges. Break apart the wedges at the fold, creating 32 chips total.

2. In a small bowl, mix the Tex-Mex seasoning and salt together.

3. Mist one side of the chips with oil, then sprinkle with half of the seasoning mix.

4. Turn the chips over, mist the other side with oil, and sprinkle with the remaining seasoning.

5. Place the pita chips in the air fryer basket and cook at 330°F for 2 minutes.

6. Shake the basket and cook for 2 more minutes.

7. Shake again and, if needed, cook for 1 or 2 more minutes, until crisp. Watch carefully to avoid burning.

NOTE: You can use either whole-grain or white pitas for this recipe, whichever you prefer.

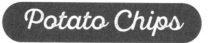

Potato Chips

Yield: 2–3 servings | Prep Time: 15 minutes | Cooking Time: 15 minutes | Total Time: 30 minutes

GLUTEN FREE   GREAT SNACK   KID FRIENDLY   TASTER FAVORITE

A mandoline makes quick work of cutting super-thin slices. A vegetable parer takes longer, but, if it's all you have, it's still worth the effort for crispy chips that taste great and are healthier too.

2 medium potatoes

2 teaspoons vegan oil

salt and pepper

oil for misting or cooking spray

1. Peel the potatoes. Peel can be left on if desired.

2. Use a mandoline or parer to shave the potatoes into very thin slices, dropping them into a bowl of water as you work.

3. Using paper towels or a clean dish towel, dry the slices thoroughly.

4. Toss the potato slices in oil to coat well.

5. Spray the air fryer basket with oil or cooking spray. Add the potatoes and stir them with a fork to separate the slices.

6. Cook at 390°F for 5 minutes.

7. Stir and break apart. Cook for 5 more minutes.

8. Stir again to separate. Cook for 5 minutes longer or until crispy.

9. Season to taste.

> **TIP:** It's normal for the centers of some of your potato chips to remain white. The edges will crisp nicely. This difference is part of the appeal of homemade chips.

Roasted Nuts

Yield: 1 cup | Prep Time: 1 minute | Cooking Time: 5–7 minutes | Total Time: 6–8 minutes

FAST   GLUTEN FREE   GREAT SNACK   SUPER EASY

We use almonds, but you can roast pecans, walnuts, and other nuts just as easily. For best results, read the notes below before you begin. The air fryer makes quick and easy work of this recipe and saves you from having to heat up your whole oven for just a small layer of food.

---

1 cup blanched whole almonds

1. Preheat the air fryer to 360°F.

2. Place the nuts in the air fryer basket.

3. Cook the nuts for 3 minutes.

4. Stop and shake the basket. Continue cooking for 2 to 4 more minutes or until the nuts brown to your liking.

> **NOTE:** Total cooking time will vary slightly depending on the type and freshness of your nuts. Watch carefully to avoid burning. After the first 3 minutes, keep checking at 1-minute intervals.
>
> **TIP:** Spread the nuts in a single layer for even cooking. Some air fryer baskets are large enough to hold more than 1 cup in a single layer.

Smoky Sandwich

Yield: 2 sandwiches | Prep Time: 5 minutes | Cooking Time: 5–8 minutes | Total Time: 10–13 minutes

FAST GREAT SNACK SUPER EASY TASTER FAVORITE

The smoky goodness of this sandwich seriously wowed our tasting panel. We think that you'll like it too.

4 slices whole-grain bread

4 slices provolone-style vegan cheese

2 slices meatless hickory-smoked deli slices

olive oil for misting

1. Lay 2 slices of bread on a cutting board.

2. On each slice of bread, layer 1 slice of vegan cheese, one deli slice, the other cheese slice, then top with the other slice of bread.

3. Mist both sides of the sandwich with oil.

4. Cut each sandwich into rectangular halves.

5. Place in the air fryer basket and cook at 390°F for 5 to 8 minutes, until the bread toasts.

TIP: We recommend Ezekiel 4:9 bread for this recipe.

VARIATION: Without the deli slices, this becomes a quick and easy grilled cheese sandwich.

Spinach-Artichoke Dip

Yield: 2 cups | Prep Time: 17 minutes | Cooking Time: 10–12 minutes | Total Time: 27–29 minutes

GLUTEN FREE   GREAT SNACK   SUPER EASY

When this recipe is done cooking, we like to wrap a pretty napkin around the baking pan and set the whole thing down in a woven basket. Add small slices of baguette toast, your favorite crackers, and a beverage and you have the perfect snack for movie night.

1 cup frozen spinach

1/3 cup vegan sour cream

1/4 cup vegan mayonnaise

1 tablespoon fresh squeezed lime juice

3 tablespoons thinly sliced green onions

3 tablespoons grated Parmesan-style topping

1 cup chopped canned artichoke hearts

oil for misting or cooking spray

small toasts or crackers for serving

1. Thaw the spinach, drain it, and squeeze out the excess moisture.

2. In a medium bowl, mix together the vegan sour cream, vegan mayonnaise, and lime juice.

3. Stir in green onions, Parmesan topping, spinach, and artichoke hearts and mix thoroughly to combine.

4. Mist the baking pan with oil or cooking spray and spoon the mixture into the baking pan.

5. Cook at 360°F for 10 to 12 minutes, until the dip heats through.

6. Serve the dip warm with small toasts or crackers.

TIP: The spinach should be thawed completely. If it's still frozen in the middle, let it sit in hot water until it completely thaws—and remember to squeeze out all the excess water before continuing with the recipe.

String Bean Fries

Yield: 4 servings | Prep Time: 15 minutes | Cooking Time: 5–6 minutes | Total Time: 20–21 minutes

GREAT SNACK

Is there a dip that doesn't taste good with these fries? If there is, we haven't found it! We've tried hot creole mustard, horseradish mayo, ranch dressing, and of course ketchup.

½ pound fresh string beans

2 tablespoons Bob's Red Mill egg replacer

½ cup water

½ cup white flour

½ cup crushed panko breadcrumbs

¼ teaspoon salt

¼ teaspoon ground black pepper

¼ teaspoon dry mustard

oil for misting or cooking spray

1. Preheat the air fryer to 360°F.

2. Trim the stem ends of the green beans, wash them, and pat them dry.

3. In a shallow dish, whisk together the egg replacer and water until well blended.

4. In a second shallow dish, place the flour.

5. In a third shallow dish, stir together the breadcrumbs, salt, pepper, and dry mustard.

6. One at a time, dip each string bean in egg mixture, flour, egg mixture again, then breadcrumbs.

7. When you've coated all the string beans, open the air fryer and place them in the basket.

8. Cook for 3 minutes.

9. Mist with oil and cook for 2 to 3 more minutes or until the string beans brown and become crispy.

TIP: If the egg wash thickens too much as you work, whisk in a little extra water to thin it.

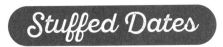

Stuffed Dates

Yield: 12 large dates | Prep Time: 15 minutes | Cooking Time: 4–5 minutes | Total Time: 19–20 minutes

GREAT SNACK   **TASTER FAVORITE**

Dates are always a great healthy choice for a sweet snack, and our stuffing takes them to a whole new level. They taste decadent but have no added sweetener.

$4\frac{1}{2}$ teaspoons Bob's Red Mill egg replacer, divided

5 tablespoons water, divided

12 large Medjool dates

$\frac{1}{4}$ cup sliced almonds

$\frac{1}{4}$ cup shredded unsweetened coconut

$\frac{1}{4}$ teaspoon almond extract

2 tablespoons cornstarch

$\frac{1}{2}$ cup crushed panko breadcrumbs

oil for misting or cooking spray

1. In a small bowl, whisk together $1\frac{1}{2}$ teaspoons of the egg replacer and 2 tablespoons of the water and set aside.

2. In each date, cut a lengthwise slit, remove the pit, and spread the date open slightly.

3. In a food processor, combine the nuts, coconut, almond extract, and 1 tablespoon of egg wash. Process in short pulses just enough to chop the nuts finely and combine the ingredients.

4. To the remaining egg wash, add the other 3 teaspoons of egg replacer and 3 tablespoons of water. Whisk to mix well.

5. Place the cornstarch in a shallow dish and the breadcrumbs in another shallow dish.

6. Preheat the air fryer to 390°F.

7. Stuff each date with the nut mixture, pressing in tightly. Overfill the dates so that the slits remain slightly open.

8. Dip each date in cornstarch, tapping off any excess.

9. Dip each date in the egg wash and then roll in the crumbs.

10. Mist the dates with oil, place them in the air fryer basket, and cook for 3 minutes.

11. Mist them with oil again and cook for 1 to 2 more minutes or until the coating browns and becomes crispy.

Sweet Potato Fries

Yield: 3–4 servings | Prep Time: 15 minutes | Cooking Time: 10–15 minutes | Total Time: 25–30 minutes

GLUTEN FREE   GREAT SNACK   KID FRIENDLY   SUPER EASY

We like to sprinkle these tasty fries with coarse sea salt, but, in a nod to Thanksgiving, you may prefer them with a sprinkle of cinnamon sugar. Either way, these are a delicious side to a burger or sandwich.

3 large sweet potatoes

1 tablespoon light olive oil

1 tablespoon dried tarragon

salt and pepper

cinnamon sugar (optional)

1. Cut the sweet potatoes into fries, $1/4$ x 3 inches. (Peeling the potatoes is optional.)

2. Toss the fries, oil, and tarragon together and stir to coat completely.

3. Pour the fries into the air fryer basket and cook at 390°F for 5 minutes.

4. Stir or shake the basket and cook for 5 more minutes, until the fries brown.

5. Season to taste with salt and pepper or cinnamon sugar.

Texas Toothpicks

Yield: 4 servings | Prep Time: 25 minutes | Cooking Time: 12–14 minutes | Total Time: 37–39 minutes

GREAT SNACK   TASTER FAVORITE

Stripping the seeds and membranes removes the hottest of the heat from jalapeños, so even the faint of heart can enjoy this classic southern treat.

1 pound jalapeño peppers

$\frac{1}{2}$ cup all-purpose white flour

$\frac{1}{2}$ cup crushed panko breadcrumbs

$\frac{1}{2}$ teaspoon smoked paprika

$\frac{1}{2}$ teaspoon onion powder

$\frac{1}{2}$ teaspoon salt

$\frac{1}{2}$ cup potato starch

$\frac{1}{2}$ cup almond milk

oil for misting or cooking spray

1. Wearing food-grade gloves, wash the jalapeños and cut them in half lengthwise.

2. Remove the seeds, membranes, and stems.

3. Cut them into long slivers about $\frac{1}{4}$-inch at the widest part.

4. Preheat the air fryer to 390°F.

5. In a plastic bag or a container with lid, combine the flour, breadcrumbs, paprika, onion powder, and salt. Shake to mix well.

6. Place the potato starch in one shallow dish and the almond milk in another.

7. Working with about a third of them at a time, dredge the pepper strips in the potato starch to coat them.

8. Shake off the excess starch and dip them in the milk, letting the excess drip off.

9. Drop the jalapeño slivers in the breadcrumbs, shake to coat, and lay them out on a cookie sheet or baking sheet.

10. When you've coated all the slivers, mist them with oil.

11. To cook the slivers all at once, make crisscross layers in the air fryer basket so that air can circulate and the strips won't stick together. Cook for 5 minutes.

12. Shake or stir gently and mist with oil. Cook for 5 more minutes.

13. Stir again, mist any remaining white spots, and cook for 2 to 4 more minutes or until the slivers turn golden brown.

Tomato-Caprese Cups

Yield: 15 pieces | Prep Time: 12 minutes | Cooking Time: 5 minutes | Total Time: 17 minutes

GREAT SNACK   SUPER EASY

These are an easy appetizer for any kind of gathering. If you have fresh basil, use that in place of the dried basil.

1 cup mozzarella-style shreds

1 (15-count) package mini phyllo cups

1½ tablespoons dried basil

15 slices black olives

8 small grape tomatoes

oil for misting

1. Coarsely chop the vegan mozzarella shreds and press into the phyllo cups, dividing evenly.

2. Sprinkle the basil over the cheese.

3. Top each with 1 black olive slice.

4. Halve the tomatoes lengthwise.

5. Place 1 tomato half cut-side down in each cup.

6. Mist the cups with oil.

7. Place the cups in the air fryer basket. You should have room to fit them all in a single layer.

8. Cook at 390°F for 5 minutes to melt the cheese.

9. Serve warm.

See insert A6 for recipe photo.

NOTE: You'll have one leftover grape tomato half—for good luck!

Tortilla Strips

Yield: 4 servings | Prep Time: 5 minutes | Cooking Time: 5–7 minutes | Total Time: 10–12 minutes

FAST GLUTEN FREE GREAT SNACK SUPER EASY

Sprinkle these crispy strips over hot soup or salads or use them as the base for your favorite salsa, dip, or snack.

---

10 (6- to 8-inch) corn tortillas

oil for misting

1. Mist each tortilla, front and back, with oil and stack.

2. Cut the tortillas into $\frac{1}{4}$ x $1\frac{1}{2}$-inch strips.

3. Place all the strips in the air fryer basket and cook at 390°F for 5 minutes.

4. Stir and cook for 2 more minutes, until they brown and become crispy.

Tuscan Tomato Toast

Yield: 2 toasts | Prep Time: 5 minutes | Cooking Time: 5–8 minutes | Total Time: 10–18 minutes

FAST GREAT SNACK SUPER EASY

Tuscan Tomato Toast is a tasty side for when your main dish is a salad (page 113), and the Tuscan Herb Mix turns tomatoes into delicious homemade marinara sauce.

1 1/2 teaspoons extra-virgin olive oil

1 teaspoon Tuscan Herb Mix (page 161)

2 slices Italian-style bread, cut to 1/2 x 3 x 6 inches

1/3–1/2 cup sundried tomatoes, coarsely chopped or torn

1 slice vegan provolone cheese

1. In a small bowl, stir the olive oil and Tuscan Herb Mix together.

2. Brush the seasoned oil on one side of the bread.

3. Cover the surface of each unoiled side of bread with the sundried tomatoes and top with cheese.

4. Cook at 390°F for 5–8 minutes, until the bottom of bread has toasted and the cheese has melted.

MAIN DISHES

Bell Peppers Stuffed with Hopping John

Yield: 3 servings | Prep Time: 22 minutes | Cooking Time: 10 minutes | Total Time: 32 minutes

GLUTEN FREE   TASTER FAVORITE

Black-eyed peas bring luck, so we southerners traditionally serve Hopping John—a mixture of black-eyed peas, rice, and sausage—on New Year's Eve. For financial fortune in the coming year, serve these peppers with a side of turnip or mustard greens or a cabbage slaw.

3 bell peppers

1 cup cooked black-eyed peas

1 cup cooked brown rice

$\frac{1}{4}$ cup minced onion

1 tablespoon Cajun Seasoning Mix (page 150)

1 tablespoon smoked paprika

salt and pepper

1. Cut about $\frac{1}{2}$ inch off the stem end of the bell peppers to create a cap and set aside.

2. Scoop out the seeds and ribs and discard.

3. In a saucepan, place the peppers and cover them with water.

4. Bring the water to boiling and boil for 5 minutes.

5. Carefully remove the peppers from the water and rinse them with cool tap water.

6. In a small bowl, mix together the peas, rice, onion, Cajun seasoning, and smoked paprika.

7. Taste for seasoning and add salt and pepper if needed.

8. Spoon the filling into the shells.

9. Replace the reserved pepper caps and place in the air fryer basket.

10. Cook at 360°F for 10 minutes.

See insert A7 for recipe photo.

TIP: When cooking black-eyed peas or brown rice, make a large batch and store extra in the freezer for when you want a simple, no-fuss meal like this. Just defrost, and you're ready to go!

VARIATION: For extra color, select 1 green, yellow, and red bell pepper each for this recipe.

Black Bean Burgers

Yield: 4 servings | Prep Time: 15 minutes | Cooking Time: 15 minutes | Total Time: 30 minutes

GLUTEN FREE

Serve these burgers on a bun, or go breadless and top them with sliced tomatoes, jalapeño peppers, and cheese-style shreds. Guacamole (page 153) also makes for a tasty topper.

---

2 (15-ounce) cans black beans, drained and rinsed

½ cup cooked quinoa

½ cup shredded sweet potato

¼ cup chopped red onion

2 teaspoons ground cumin

1 teaspoon ground coriander seed

½ teaspoon salt

oil for misting or cooking spray

1. In a medium bowl, mash the beans with a fork or potato masher.

2. Add the quinoa, sweet potato, onion, cumin, coriander, and salt and stir until well mixed.

3. Shape the mixture into 4 patties, about ¾-inch thick.

4. Mist both sides of the patties with oil or cooking spray.

5. Spray the air fryer basket with oil or cooking spray, add the bean burgers, and cook at 390°F for 15 minutes.

Bread Pockets

Yield: 4 servings | Prep Time: 10 minutes | Cooking Time: 8–10 minutes | Total Time: 18–20 minutes

Choose your own adventure here: Italian-style for dipping into pizza sauce or muffuletta-style. The recipe below adapts a standard pepperoni pocket into a hearty vegan meal, but you can fill the pocket with any of your favorite veggies and spreads, including artichoke hearts, avocados, onions, peppers, hummus, pesto, tapenade, etc. However you slice it, our favorite bread for this recipe is a ready-to-bake artisan loaf—but plain French or Italian bread also will work.

---

4 thick bread slices, 1-inch thick

olive oil for misting

4 heaping tablespoons chopped mushrooms

¼ cup chopped black olives

4 tablespoons mozzarella or Monterey Jack & Cheddar–style shreds

pizza sauce (optional)

1. Mist both sides of the bread slices with oil.

2. Stand the slices upright and cut a cavity in the bread from the top, making a deep pocket. Cut almost to the bottom crust, taking care not to cut through the sides or through the bottom.

3. Into each bread pocket, place chopped mushrooms, a tablespoon of olives, and a heaping tablespoon of cheese-style shreds.

4. Stand the bread pockets upright in the air fryer basket.

5. Cook at 360°F for 8 to 10 minutes, until the filling is hot and the bread has browned.

6. Serve hot, with pizza or other sauce for dipping if you like.

> **VARIATION:** Spicy Bread Pocket: Before filling, spread coarse brown mustard inside the pockets. Omit black olives and use chopped green olives instead. Cook as directed above and serve hot with extra mustard for dipping.

Brown Rice Bake

Yield: 2–4 servings | Prep Time: 4 minutes | Cooking Time: 6–8 minutes | Total Time: 10–12 minutes

GLUTEN FREE   SUPER EASY   TASTER FAVORITE

In larger servings, this satisfying recipe works great as a main dish. It also makes a delicious side for a summer picnic or other outing.

1 teaspoon sesame oil

⅓ cup chopped onion

⅓ cup chopped bell pepper

2 cups cooked brown rice

1 (8-ounce) can crushed pineapple, drained

½ teaspoon salt

1. In the baking pan, place the oil, onion, and bell pepper, cook for 1 minute, and stir.

2. Cook the veggie mixture for 3 to 4 more minutes or just until the vegetables become tender.

3. Transfer the vegetables to a bowl and add the rice, pineapple, and salt, stirring until well mixed.

4. Pour the mixture back into the air fryer baking pan and cook at 390°F for 2 to 3 minutes, until everything heats through.

TIP: Serve Sriracha sauce for those who want a fiery-hot version of this dish.

VARIATIONS: To give this recipe more tropical flair, stir in ¼ cup of shredded coconut at the end and top with chopped macadamias, Brazils, or other nuts.

To make this a heartier dish, add 1 cup of cooked, crumbled seitan (in step 3).

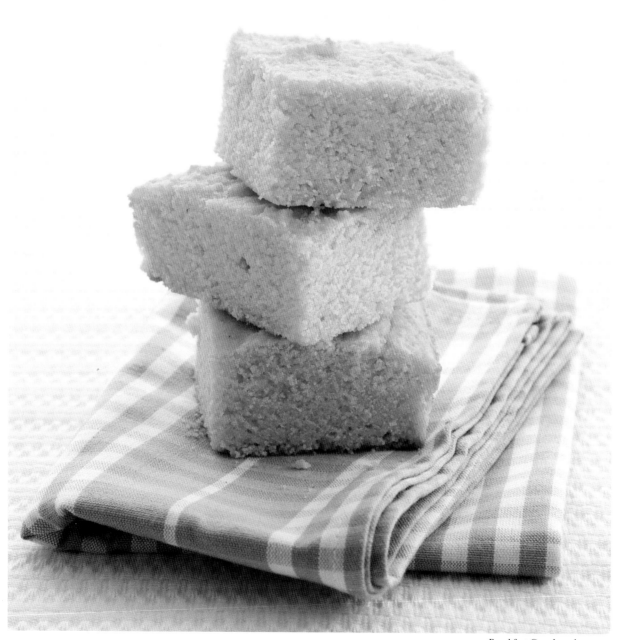

Breakfast Cornbread, page 2

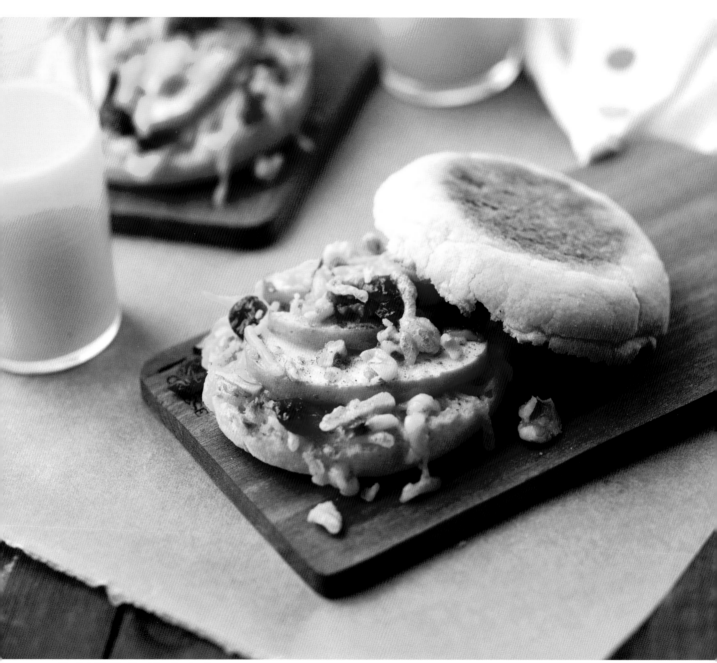

English Muffin Breakfast Sandwich, page 5

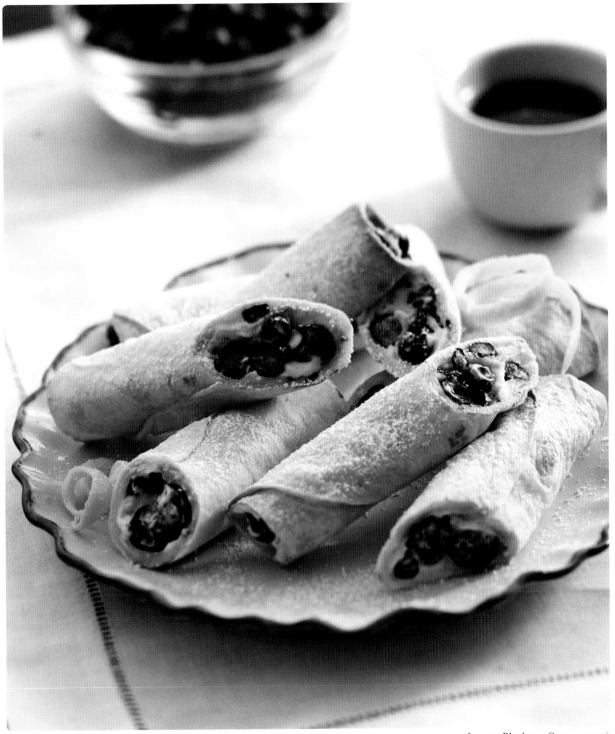

Lemon-Blueberry Crepes, page 7

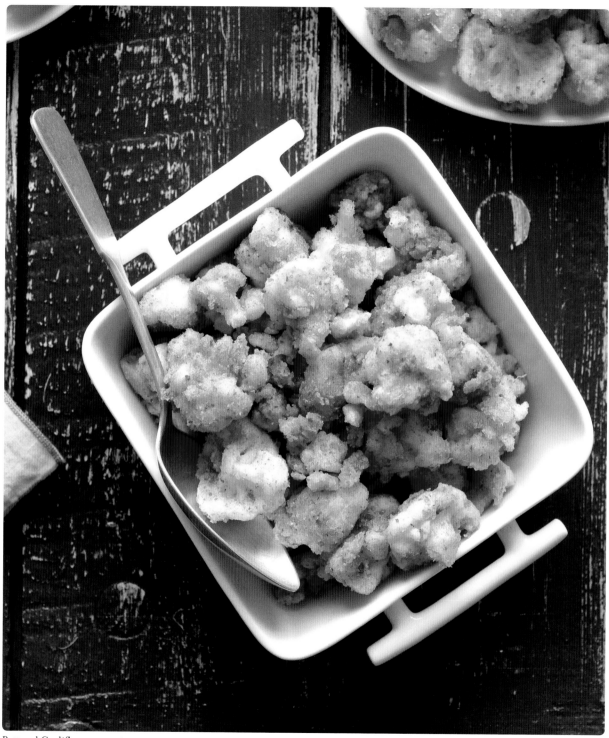

Battered Cauliflower, page 23

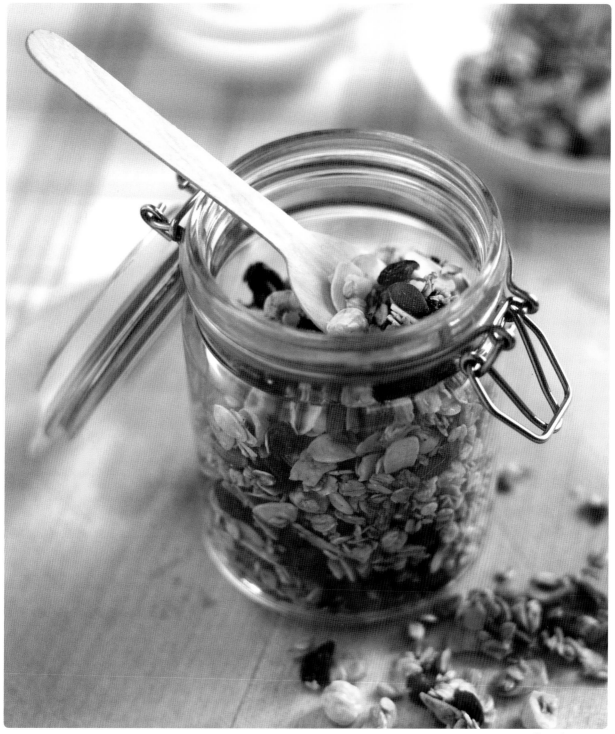

Granola, page 32

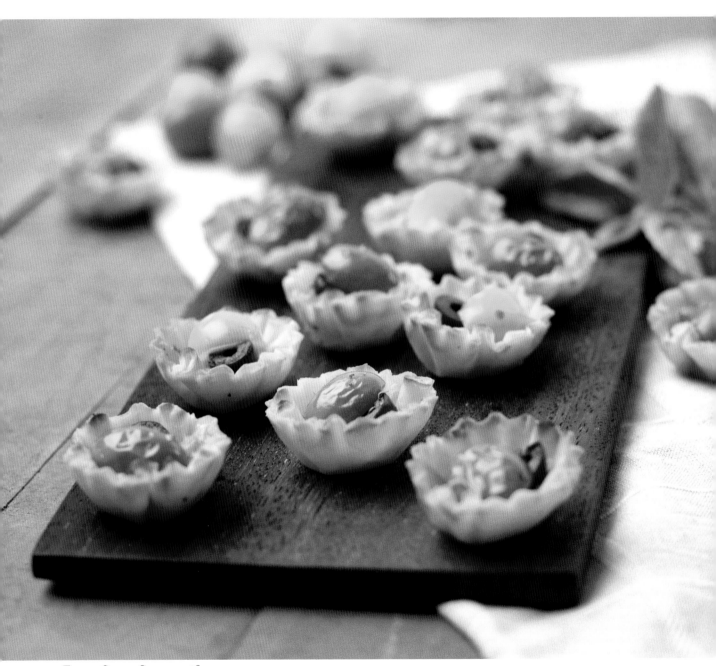

Tomato-Caprese Cups, page 46

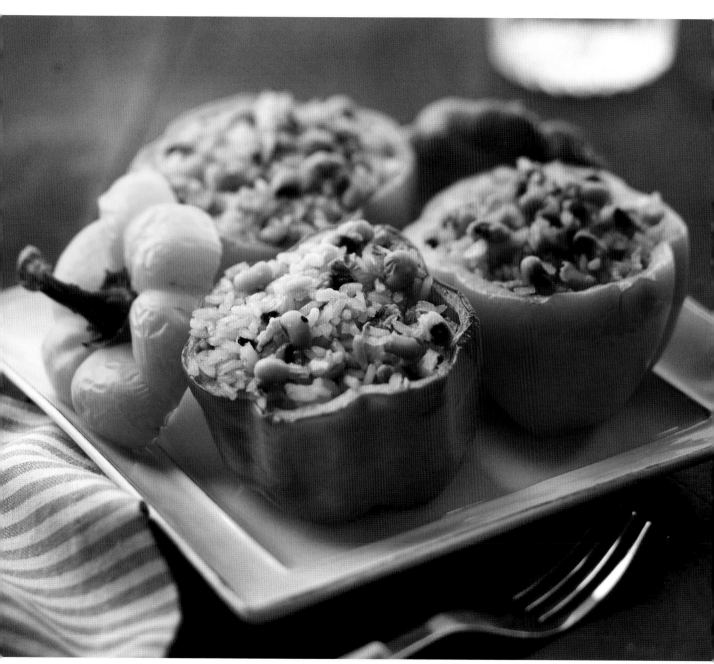

Bell Peppers Stuffed with Hopping John, page 51

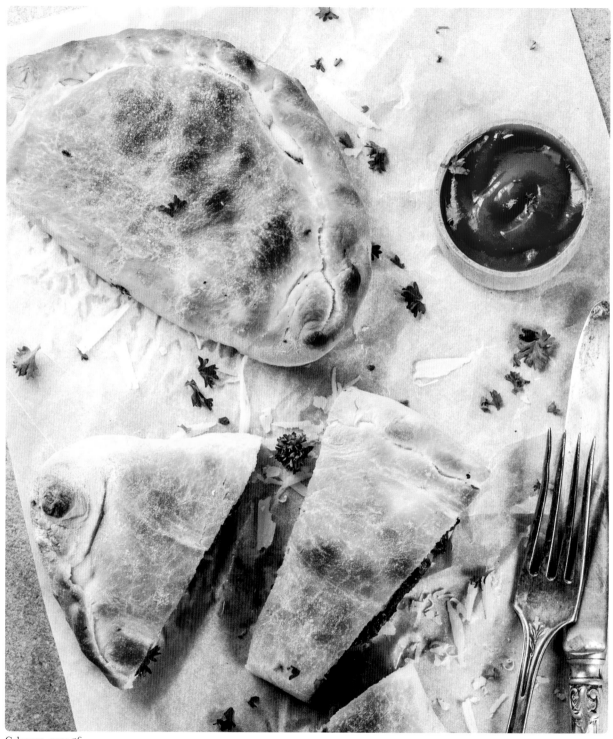

Calzones, page 56

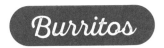

Burritos

Yield: 4 servings | Prep Time: 12 minutes | Cooking Time: 10 minutes | Total Time: 22 minutes

KID FRIENDLY

If you have flour tortillas on hand, you can pull this quick meal together from your pantry in almost no time. Serve this family favorite with shredded lettuce on the side, topped with Guacamole (page 153) or Pico de Gallo (page 156).

1 cup vegan refried beans

1 tablespoon Tex-Mex Seasoning (page 159)

4 (10-inch) flour tortillas

½ cup sliced black olives

½ cup drained and sliced jalapeños (from a small jar)

1 cup Cheddar-style shreds

1. In a small bowl, mix together the beans and seasoning.
2. On each tortilla, place ¼ cup of beans about 2 inches from the edge.
3. Top the beans with a quarter of the olives, jalapeños, and cheese.
4. Fold the nearest tortilla edge over the filling and roll 1 turn.
5. Fold in each side and finish rolling up.
6. Place 2 burritos in the air fryer basket, seam side down.
7. Lay the other 2 burritos on top of the first two, crosswise, seam side down.
8. Cook at 390°F for 5 minutes.
9. Rearrange the burritos so that you switch the top and bottom layers.
10. Cook for 5 more minutes or until the burritos slightly brown and heat through.

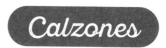

Calzones

Yield: 8 calzones | Prep Time: 20 minutes | Cooking Time: 7–8 minutes per batch (2 batches) | Total Time: 34–36 minutes

Using rapid-rise yeast enables you to get these traditional calzones on the table in short order. For a different twist, check out the Calzones Tex-Mex (page 57).

Crust

2 cups white wheat flour, plus more for kneading and rolling

1 (¼-ounce) package rapid-rise yeast

1 teaspoon salt

½ teaspoon dried basil

1 cup warm water (115–125°F)

2 teaspoons extra-light olive oil

Filling

½ cup sliced mushrooms

oil for misting or cooking spray

2 links vegan Italian sausage (about 7 ounces)

½ cup chopped red bell pepper

½ cup chopped green bell pepper

¼ teaspoon dried basil

¼ teaspoon garlic powder

¼ teaspoon ground oregano

½ teaspoon dried parsley

1⅓ cups Monterey Jack & Cheddar–style shreds

2 tablespoons grated Parmesan-style topping

marinara sauce (optional)

See insert A8 for recipe photo.

1. First make the crust. In a medium bowl, combine the flour, yeast, salt, basil, warm water, and oil.

2. Stir until a soft dough forms.

3. Turn the dough out onto a lightly floured board and knead for 3 or 4 minutes.

4. Let the dough rest for 10 minutes.

5. Next make the filling. Place the mushrooms in the air fryer baking pan, mist them with oil, and cook at 390°F for 2 minutes.

6. Meanwhile, cut the vegan sausage into thin slices. Add the vegan sausage slices to the mushrooms.

7. Stir in the red and green bell pepper, garlic, oregano, basil, and parsley and cook for 3 minutes.

8. Stir and continue cooking for 3 more minutes or until the vegetables are crisp-tender.

9. Remove the pan from the air fryer. Stir in both vegan cheeses and set aside to cool.

10. Divide the dough into 8 portions. Working with 4 pieces of the dough per batch, press each into a 6-inch circle.

11. Divide half of the filling mixture into the 4 dough circles.

12. Fold each circle over to create a half-moon shape.

13. Press the edges together, sealing them firmly to prevent any leakage.

14. Spray both sides of the 4 calzones with oil or cooking spray, place them in the air fryer basket, and cook at 360°F for 5 minutes.

15. Mist the calzones with oil or spray again and cook them for 2 to 3 more minutes, until the crust has browned nicely.

16. Shape and fill the remaining 4 calzones and cook as above.

17. Top with marinara sauce or serve with the marinara sauce on the side for dipping.

Calzones Tex-Mex

Yield: 8 calzones | Prep Time: 20 minutes | Cooking Time: 7–8 minutes per batch (2 batches) | Total Time: 34–36 minutes

We think Tex-Mex tastes great, but it can be too hot for some people. A good way to please different palates with this recipe is to omit the jalapeño from the filling and add it to the salsa or Pico de Gallo instead. Just make sure to reserve some of the mild salsa or Pico for anyone who isn't crazy about crazy hot.

Crust

2 cups white wheat flour, plus more for kneading and rolling

1 (1/4-ounce) package rapid-rise yeast

1 teaspoon salt

1 cup warm water (115–125°F)

2 teaspoons extra-light olive oil

Filling

1/4 cup finely chopped onion

1 jalapeño, seeded and chopped (optional)

1/2 cup cooked pinto beans

1/4 cup cooked corn kernels

1/2 (4 1/2-ounce) can chopped green chile peppers

1 teaspoon chili powder

1/8 teaspoon oregano

1/4 teaspoon garlic powder

1/4 teaspoon onion powder

1/4 teaspoon cumin

1/2 cup Monterey Jack & Cheddar–style shreds

salt

oil for misting or cooking spray

1 tablespoon yellow cornmeal

salsa or Pico de Gallo (page 156) for serving

1. First make the crust. In a medium bowl, combine the flour, yeast, and salt.
2. Stir in the warm water and oil until a soft dough forms.
3. On a lightly floured board, knead the dough for 3 or 4 minutes.
4. Let the dough rest for about 10 minutes.
5. Place the chopped onion and jalapeño in the baking pan and mist with oil or cooking spray. Cook at 390°F for 2 to 4 minutes until tender, stirring halfway through.
6. Place the onion mixture in a medium bowl and stir in the remaining filling ingredients.
7. Divide the dough into 8 portions.
8. Working with 4 pieces of the dough at a time, press each into a 6-inch circle.
9. Divide half of the filling mixture evenly among the 4 dough circles.
10. Fold each circle over to create a half-moon shape. Press the edges together and seal firmly to prevent leakage.
11. Spray both sides of the calzone with oil or cooking spray and dust the tops lightly with cornmeal.
12. Place 4 calzones in the air fryer basket and cook at 360°F for 5 minutes.
13. Mist them with oil or spray and cook for 2 to 3 more minutes, until the crust nicely browns.
14. Shape and fill the remaining 4 calzones and cook as directed above.
15. Serve with plenty of salsa or Pico de Gallo (page 156) on the side—or both!

Chickenless Parmesan

Yield: 2 servings | Prep Time: 5 minutes | Cooking Time: 20–25 minutes | Total Time: 25–30 minutes

SUPER EASY   TASTER FAVORITE

You can cook this tasty meal quite quickly. Put the water on to boil for the angel hair and start the patties. By the time the pasta is done, the patties will be ready.

4 ounces angel hair pasta

2 breaded chicken-style patties

2 teaspoons grated Parmesan-style topping

½ cup spaghetti or marinara sauce, plus 2 tablespoons, divided

1. Cook the angel hair pasta according to the package directions.

2. While waiting for the water to boil, put the patties in the air fryer basket.

3. Cook the patties at 390°F for 10 minutes.

4. Flip the patties and top each with 1 teaspoon of the Parmesan topping.

5. Spoon 1 tablespoon of sauce over each patty and cook an additional 10 to 15 minutes, until heated through.

6. Drain the pasta and toss with the remaining ½ cup of sauce.

7. Divide the pasta between 2 bowls or plates and top with the patties.

NOTE: For this recipe, we recommend Gardein Crispy Chick'n Patties.

VARIATION: Substitute Pecan-Crusted Eggplant (page 67) for the chicken-style patties.

Chiles Rellenos

TASTER FAVORITE

Our version of a popular restaurant dish has less fat of course and doesn't taste quite so heavy. We especially like salsa verde spooned over the chiles, but use whichever salsa you prefer.

2 poblano peppers

1 cup veggie ground crumbles

¼ cup minced onion

1 teaspoon light olive oil

1 cup fresh or frozen corn kernels

1 tablespoon chili powder

1 tablespoon cocoa powder

½ teaspoon salt

Batter

½ cup all-purpose flour

1 tablespoon Bob's Red Mill egg replacer

⅛ teaspoon salt

¾ cup almond milk

Breading

1½–2 cups panko breadcrumbs

1 cup all-purpose white flour

oil for misting or cooking spray

¼ cup red or green salsa for serving

> **TIP:** The breading process is messy, and you may need to rinse your fingers so that the panko will stick to the poblanos and not to you. Food-grade gloves will help.

1. Lay the poblanos flat and cut a slit in each on one side.

2. In a small saucepan, cover the peppers with water.

3. Bring to boiling and boil for 5 minutes.

4. Remove the poblanos from the pan and rinse them with cool tap water.

5. While poblanos are boiling, prepare the filling. In a baking pan, cook the crumbles and onion in the oil at 390°F for 3 minutes.

6. Stir in the corn, chili powder, cocoa powder, and salt.

7. Stuff the filling into the peppers and close them together with toothpicks.

8. In a shallow bowl, mix all of the batter ingredients together.

9. On a sheet of wax paper, place the panko crumbs.

10. Onto another sheet of wax paper, place the flour.

11. Carefully spoon the flour around and over all sides of the stuffed poblanos.

12. Place the peppers in the bowl of batter and spoon it over them to coat all sides.

13. Dredge the battered poblanos in the panko, pressing the breadcrumbs into all sides.

14. Mist the peppers with oil, carefully set them in the air fryer basket, and cook at 390°F for 10 minutes, until they brown and become crispy.

15. Remove the toothpicks and top the poblanos with salsa just before serving.

Coconut Tofu

Yield: 4 servings | Prep Time: 40 minutes | Cooking Time: 5–6 minutes per batch (2 batches) | Total Time: 50–52 minutes

TASTER FAVORITE

Thanks to the pineapple marinade, this flavorful tofu needs no dipping sauce. Serve it alongside your favorite vegetable medley or Asian-style rice.

1 (14-ounce) block extra-firm tofu, pressed

1½ cups pineapple juice

2 tablespoons Bob's Red Mill egg replacer

¾ cup shredded coconut

¾ cup panko breadcrumbs

salt

oil for misting or cooking spray

1. Cut the tofu into ½-inch cubes.

2. Pour the pineapple juice over the tofu and marinate for 30 minutes.

3. Drain the tofu and reserve the marinating juice.

4. In a shallow dish, mix the egg replacer and ¼ cup of the reserved juice. Let it sit for 1 minute to thicken.

5. In another shallow dish, combine the coconut and breadcrumbs.

6. Sprinkle the tofu with salt to taste.

7. Preheat the air fryer to 390°F.

8. Add 3 more tablespoons of reserved pineapple juice to the egg wash and whisk until smooth.

9. Working with a few pieces at a time, dip the tofu in the egg wash and then roll it in the coconut mixture.

10. Spray the tofu chunks with oil or cooking spray and place them in the air fryer basket in a single layer, close together but not touching.

11. Cook for 5 to 6 minutes, until light golden brown.

12. Repeat steps 10 and 11 to cook the remaining tofu.

> **TIP:** If the egg wash becomes too thick as you work, add 1 more tablespoon of the reserved pineapple juice or water to thin it.

Empanadas

Yield: 8 servings | Prep Time: 30 minutes | Cooking Time: 12–22 minutes | Total Time: 42–52 minutes

These empanadas taste fairly mild, so, if you like a little more heat, feel free to add a few jalapeño slices before sealing the dough.

Filling

1 (9-ounce) package chicken-style strips

oil for misting

1 (4-ounce) can chopped green chiles, drained

¼ cup chopped sundried tomatoes

½ teaspoon cumin

½ teaspoon thyme

Dough

1 cup masa harina flour

½ cup all-purpose white flour

½ teaspoon baking powder

¼ teaspoon salt

½ cup water

¼ cup almond milk

1. First make the filling. Spray the chicken-style strips with oil and place them in the air fryer basket.

2. Cook at 360°F for 2 minutes.

3. Blot the chopped green chiles with paper towels to remove excess moisture.

4. Coarsely chop the chicken-style strips and mix with the chiles, sundried tomatoes, cumin, and thyme.

5. Next make the dough. In a medium bowl, stir together the masa harina, white flour, baking powder, and salt.

6. Stir in the water and milk to make a soft dough.

7. Divide the dough into 8 portions and then roll each into a ball.

8. Roll each ball into a 4-inch circle.

9. Divide the filling mixture evenly over the dough circles.

10. Using a finger dipped in water, moisten the edges of the circles and fold them over to make a half-moon pie.

11. Crimp the edges closed with a fork.

12. Place 4 empanadas in the fryer basket and cook at 360°F for 5 minutes.

13. Flip the empanadas over and cook for 5 to 10 more minutes, until light brown.

14. Repeat steps 12 and 13 to cook the remaining empanadas.

NOTE: For this recipe, we recommended Gardein Chick'n Strips.

Fishless Sticks with Remoulade

Yield: 2 servings | Prep Time: 5 minutes | Cooking Time: 5 minutes | Total Time: 10 minutes

FAST   GREAT SNACK   KID FRIENDLY   SUPER EASY   TASTER FAVORITE

The right sauce can improve this standby kid favorite enormously. Try our Remoulade to whip up a super-fast lunch that kids of all ages will enjoy.

1 (7.05-ounce) package frozen fishless sticks (10 count)

Remoulade

½ cup vegan mayonnaise

2 tablespoons ketchup

1 tablespoon yellow mustard

1 tablespoon tarragon vinegar

¼ medium onion, grated

salt

1. Preheat the air fryer to 390°F.

2. Place all of the fishless sticks in the air fryer basket and cook for 5 minutes or until thoroughly heated through. You don't need any extra oil for crisping.

3. While the air fryer is preheating and cooking, stir together all of the sauce ingredients.

4. Serve the fishless sticks with the Remoulade for dipping.

> **TIP:** The Remoulade also makes a good dip for the Asparagus Fries (page 19), Avocado Fries (page 20), String Bean Fries (page 42), or Sweet Potato Fries (page 44).

Italian Pita Pockets

Yield: 4 servings | Prep Time: 10 minutes | Cooking Time: 12–13 minutes | Total Time: 22–23 minutes

These pita pockets come together so quickly that they're perfect for busy weeknights. Fill with your ingredients of choice, including more peppers, mushrooms, other veggies, or vegan sausage. Don't forget to pile on your favorite vegan cheese!

2 medium green or red bell peppers

oil for misting

4 pita pocket halves

¼ cup marinara sauce

4 tablespoons mozzarella-style shreds

1. Cut the bell pepper into strips, about ¼ to ⅜-inch in width.

2. Place the pepper strips in the air fryer basket and mist them with oil.

3. Cook at 390°F for 8 minutes or until the peppers are tender.

4. Remove everything from the basket.

5. In each pita pocket, place 1 tablespoon marinara sauce, 1 heaping tablespoon of mozzarella shreds, and ¼ of the bell pepper strips.

6. Place the pita halves in the air fryer basket, standing up and leaning against the sides of the basket and one another.

7. Cook for 4 to 5 minutes at 390°F to heat through. Serve hot.

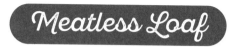

Meatless Loaf

Yield: 4 servings | Prep Time: 15 minutes | Cooking Time: 40 minutes | Total Time: 55 minutes

SUPER EASY

Our taste testers loved this loaf even without the topping. We think you'll like it either way.

Loaf

2 cups veggie ground crumbles

¼ cup minced onion

¼ cup minced zucchini

¼ cup minced sundried tomatoes

¼ cup minced green bell pepper

1 tablespoon vegan Worcestershire sauce

1 tablespoon Bob's Red Mill egg replacer

2 tablespoons water

oil for misting or cooking spray

Topping (optional)

¼ cup ketchup

1½ teaspoons vegan Worcestershire sauce

1 tablespoon blackstrap molasses

1. In a medium bowl, mix all of the loaf ingredients together.

2. Spray the baking pan with oil or cooking spray and pack the loaf down into the pan.

3. Cook at 360°F for 30 minutes.

4. While the loaf is cooking, mix all of the topping ingredients together.

5. Spoon the topping over the loaf and cook for 10 more minutes.

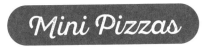

Mini Pizzas

Yield: 4 servings | Prep Time: 10 minutes | Cooking Time: 4 minutes per batch (2 batches) | Total Time: 18 minutes

GREAT SNACK KID FRIENDLY

Satisfy your pizza craving in a snap with mini pizza muffins that are ready to hit the table in fewer than 20 minutes.

2 vegan Italian sausage links (about 7 ounces)

2 English muffins

½ cup marinara sauce

¼ cup sliced ripe olives

½ cup mozzarella-style shreds

1. Preheat the air fryer to 390°F.

2. Cut each sausage in half crosswise. Then split each half lengthwise to make a total of 8 pieces.

3. Split the muffins in half.

4. On each muffin half, spread 2 tablespoons marinara sauce.

5. Top with 2 pieces of vegan sausage, leaving a little space in between the two sausage pieces.

6. Place 1 tablespoon of olives down the center of each muffin, between the sausage pieces.

7. Top each muffin with 1 heaping tablespoon of cheese shreds.

8. Place 2 mini pizzas in the air fryer basket and cook for 4 minutes or until the cheese melts and the bottoms of the muffins have crisped.

9. Repeat step 8 to cook the remaining mini pizzas.

See insert B1 for recipe photo.

> **NOTE:** If your air fryer basket will hold all 4 halves, cook them all at once. The cooking time should remain about the same.
>
> **VARIATION:** For a crispier crust, layer in this order: muffin half, cheese, vegan sausage, olives, sauce.
> Substitute any vegetable or even fruit (like pineapple) that you typically enjoy on pizza.

Mushroom-Onion Hand Pies

Yield: 8 small pies | Prep Time: 15 minutes | Cooking Time: 20 minutes | Total Time: 35 minutes

Kale adds extra nutrition and a nice crunch to these little pies. For kids or otherwise picky eaters, soften the kale by cooking it with the other filling ingredients in step 1.

Filling

1 tablespoon extra-light olive oil

1½ cups chopped mushrooms

¼ cup chopped onion

1 cup chopped kale (slightly packed)

1 tablespoon lemon juice

¼ teaspoon garlic powder

salt and pepper

Crust

1½ cups all-purpose white flour

¼ teaspoon salt

⅓ cup coconut oil (solid)

8 tablespoons cold water

oil for misting or cooking spray

1. First make the filling. Pour the oil in the baking pan, add the mushrooms and onions, and stir.

2. Cook for 5 minutes at 390°F.

3. Stir in the kale, lemon juice, garlic powder, and salt and pepper to taste. Set aside to cool.

4. Next make the crust. In a large bowl, combine the flour and salt.

5. With a pastry blender, cut in the coconut oil.

6. Add 6 tablespoons of water and stir. Continue stirring and add just enough of the remaining water to make a stiff pie dough.

7. Divide the dough into 8 portions.

8. Pat each dough portion into a circle, about 5 inches in diameter.

9. Divide the filling evenly among the dough circles.

10. Fold each dough circle into a half-moon shape and firmly crimp the edges closed with a fork.

11. Spray both sides of the hand pie with oil or cooking spray and place all 8 pies in the air fryer basket.

12. Cook at 390°F for 10 minutes.

13. If the pies aren't browning well, spray them with more oil. Cook for 5 more minutes or until the pies have browned and the crust has cooked through.

Pecan-Crusted Eggplant

Yield: 4 servings | Prep Time: 15 minutes | Cooking Time: 6–8 minutes per batch (2 batches) | Total Time: 27–31 minutes

TASTER FAVORITE

This crusty coating tastes best when it contains good-size chunks of pecans. Most food processors work very fast, so take care that you don't overdo it and end up with pecan meal.

---

2 tablespoons Bob's Red Mill egg replacer

4 tablespoons water

1 cup panko breadcrumbs

$1/4$ teaspoon salt

$1/4$ teaspoon pepper

$1/4$ teaspoon dry mustard

$1/4$ teaspoon marjoram

$1/2$ cup pecans

6 tablespoons almond milk

1 large eggplant, about $1^{1}/_{4}$ pounds

salt and pepper

oil for misting or cooking spray

1. In a medium bowl, mix the egg replacer and water together and set aside.

2. In a food processor, pulse the breadcrumbs, salt, pepper, mustard, and marjoram until you have finely crushed crumbs.

3. Add the pecans and process in short pulses until the nuts are chopped. Go easy so you don't overdo it!

4. Preheat the air fryer to 390°F.

5. Transfer the coating mixture from the food processor into a shallow dish.

6. Add the almond milk to the egg mixture and whisk to combine well.

7. Cut the eggplant into $1/2$-inch slices and sprinkle with salt and pepper to taste.

8. Dip the eggplant slices in the milk wash, then roll in the crumbs, pressing to coat them well.

9. Spray both sides of each slice with oil.

10. Place half of the eggplant slices in the air fryer basket (see the note at left) and cook for 6 to 8 minutes or until the coating turns golden brown and crispy.

11. Repeat step 10 to cook the remaining slices.

See insert B2 for recipe photo.

NOTE: Don't stack the eggplant slices in the air fryer basket. It's OK to lean them against the sides of the basket so that you can fit more slices in each batch, though. If you're unsure about placement, remember that the point is to leave enough space for hot air to flow around the food.

Poblano Enchiladas

Yield: 3–4 servings | Prep Time: 29 minutes | Cooking Time: 20 minutes | Total Time: 49 minutes

GLUTEN FREE   TASTER FAVORITE

Poblano peppers add a nice bite to these enchiladas without leaving the burn. You don't need to press the tofu for this recipe.

Vegetable Sauté

1 tablespoon light olive oil

¹/₂ cup diced zucchini (¹/₄-inch dice)

¹/₄ cup diced onion (¹/₄-inch dice)

¹/₄ cup diced poblano pepper (¹/₄-inch dice)

Enchilada

¹/₄ cup mashed avocado

1 (7-ounce) can salsa verde

³/₄ cup firm tofu, diced into ¹/₄-inch pieces

8–10 (5- or 6-inch diameter) corn tortillas

1. Into the air fryer baking pan, add the olive oil, zucchini, onion, and poblano pepper.

2. Cook at 390°F for 5 minutes, until the vegetables become tender.

3. Pour the vegetables into a small bowl, set aside, and return the baking pan to the air fryer.

4. In another small bowl, stir the mashed avocado and 2 tablespoons of the salsa verde together.

5. Add the avocado mixture and tofu cubes to the bowl of vegetables and stir to combine.

6. Spoon 1 tablespoon of the filling down one side of each tortilla and then roll it up.

7. Place four of the rolled tortillas in the baking pan and spoon 1¹/₂ teaspoons of the salsa verde over each one.

8. Stack the remaining 4 tortillas on the ones in the baking pan and spoon the remainder of the salsa verde over them.

9. Cook at 360°F for 15 minutes.

Polenta Half-Moons with Creole Sauce

Yield: 4–5 servings | Prep Time: 21 minutes | Cooking Time: 15–30 minutes | Total Time: 36–51 minutes

The Creole sauce in this recipe might taste a bit spicy for some palates. If that's the case, simply reduce the amount of seasoning to lower the heat level. The frozen mirepoix perks up a pot of beans.

Creole Sauce

1 (14-ounce) bag frozen mirepoix

1 (4-ounce) can chopped mushrooms, drained

1–2 tablespoons Cajun Seasoning Mix (page 150)

1 tablespoon water

Polenta Half-Moons

1 cup all-purpose white flour

½ cup almond milk

2 cups panko breadcrumbs

1 (18-ounce) roll polenta

oil for misting or cooking spray

1. In the baking pan, stir together all the ingredients for the sauce and cook at 360°F for 5 minutes.

2. Stir, cook for 5 more minutes, and set aside.

3. While the sauce is cooking, set up your breading station: flour on a sheet of wax paper, milk in a shallow bowl, and breadcrumbs on another sheet of wax paper.

4. Cut the polenta into ½-inch slices.

5. Dredge the polenta discs in the flour, then milk, and finally breadcrumbs. On a cutting board, lay each slice and cut in half to create a half-moon shape.

6. Mist all sides of the half-moons with oil or cooking spray and stand half of the slices in the air fryer, close together but not touching.

7. Cook at 390°F for 15 minutes, until lightly brown and crisp.

8. Repeat step 7 with the remaining half-moon slices.

9. To serve, spoon 1 tablespoon of the Creole Sauce over each half-moon.

> **NOTE:** Mirepoix, a staple of French cooking, consists of diced carrots, celery, and onions. Most grocery stores carry it fresh in the vegetable or deli department or frozen. If yours doesn't, you can make your own: ⅓ cup of each ingredient would suffice for this recipe.

Savory Corn Muffins

Yield: 10 muffins | Prep Time: 12 minutes | Cooking Time: 2–3 minutes seeds, 12–13 minutes
muffins per batch (2 batches) | Total Time: 38–41 minutes

Enjoy the cozy fall flavor of these muffins with Squash Casserole (page 107) or Root Vegetables (page 106). They also go great with your favorite hot soup.

1 tablespoon flaxseed meal

2 tablespoons water

10 foil muffin cups

cooking spray

3/4 cup flour

1 cup yellow cornmeal

2 1/2 teaspoons baking powder

1/2 teaspoon salt

1/4 teaspoon rubbed sage

1/4 teaspoon ground marjoram

1/4 teaspoon ground black pepper

1/2 teaspoon rubbed thyme

1/8 teaspoon ground nutmeg

1/4 cup raw pumpkin seeds

1/2 cup almond milk

2 tablespoons extra light olive oil

3/4 cup canned pumpkin

1/4 cup cooked corn kernels, drained

1/4 cup black beans, drained

1. Mix flaxseed and water in a medium bowl and set aside.

2. Remove paper liners from foil muffin cups and save for another use. Spray the foil cups lightly with cooking spray.

3. Preheat the air fryer to 390°F.

4. In large bowl stir together flour, cornmeal, baking powder, salt, sage, marjoram, pepper, thyme, and nutmeg.

5. Place pumpkin seeds in the air fryer baking pan. Cook at 390°F for 2 minutes. Shake the pan and, if needed, cook up to a minute longer until lightly toasted.

6. While pumpkin seeds cook, add almond milk, olive oil, and pumpkin to a bowl with the prepared flaxseed water. Stir until well combined.

7. Pour the liquid mixture into the bowl with the dry ingredients. Add the corn, beans, and seeds. Stir just until moistened. Do not beat. Batter will be very thick.

8. Spoon the mixture into prepared muffin cups, dividing evenly.

9. Place 5 muffin cups in the air fryer basket. Cook at 390°F for 12 to 13 minutes or until a toothpick inserted in the center of a muffin comes out clean.

10. Repeat step 9 to bake the remaining muffins.

> **TIP:** Looking for a way to use up the rest of that can of pumpkin? Use in the variation for Flourless Oat Muffins on page 6.

Seitan Nuggets

Yield: 2–3 servings | Prep Time: 15 minutes | Cooking Time: 8–9 minutes | Total Time: 23–24 minutes

GREAT SNACK

Seitan is pure wheat protein or gluten. Hearty eaters may get only 2 servings from this recipe, but you can double the amounts easily. Follow the directions below but cook in two batches.

2 teaspoons Bob's Red Mill egg replacer

4 tablespoons water

Seasoning

$^1/_2$ teaspoon salt

$^1/_4$ teaspoon oregano

$1^1/_4$ teaspoons celery seed

$1^1/_4$ teaspoons ground mustard

$^1/_4$ teaspoon paprika

$^1/_2$ teaspoon garlic powder

$^1/_2$ teaspoon dried basil, crushed

$^1/_4$ teaspoon black pepper

$^1/_4$ teaspoon ground ginger

$^3/_4$ cup panko breadcrumbs

2 tablespoons potato starch

1 (8-ounce) package seitan strips, traditional flavor

oil for misting or cooking spray

1. In a shallow dish, mix the egg replacer and water together and set aside.

2. In a small cup, stir together all of the seasoning ingredients.

3. In another shallow dish, stir together the breadcrumbs and $2^1/_2$ teaspoons of the seasoning mix.

4. Place the potato starch in a plastic bag or a container with a lid.

5. Preheat the air fryer to 390°F.

6. Gently separate the seitan strips and sprinkle them with the remaining seasoning mix.

7. Place the seasoned seitan strips in the bag or container with the potato starch and shake to coat.

8. Working with a few pieces at a time, dip the seitan strips in the egg wash, then roll them in the seasoned crumbs.

9. When you've coated all the strips, spray them with oil, place them in the air fryer basket, and cook them for 5 minutes.

10. Shake the basket to redistribute the nuggets and mist them with oil again.

11. Cook 3 to 4 more minutes or until the nuggets become crispy and golden brown.

Sweet Potato Empanadas

Yield: 8 empanadas | Prep Time: 22 minutes | Cooking Time: 5–8 minutes | Total Time: 27–30 minutes

GREAT SNACK TASTER FAVORITE

When our tasting panel tasted these savory turnovers, they asked us to make a second batch. They're that good!

⅓ cup cooked mashed sweet potato

¼ cup cooked quinoa

1 tablespoon minced green onions

2 tablespoons chopped roasted peanuts

½ teaspoon curry powder

8 (4-inch diameter) flour tortillas

oil for misting

1. In a small bowl, mix the sweet potato, quinoa, onion, peanuts, and curry powder.

2. Place 1 tablespoon of the filling in the center of each tortilla.

3. Using your finger or the back of a spoon, moisten the edge of the tortilla all around with water.

4. Fold the tortilla in half to make a half-moon shape. Press the center gently to distribute the filling, then press the edges firmly to seal.

5. Spray both sides of each empanada with oil.

6. Place the empanadas in the air fryer basket, close together but not overlapping.

7. Cook at 390°F for 5–8 minutes, just until the empanadas have browned lightly and are crispy.

Tofu in Hoisin Sauce

Yield: 2 servings | Prep Time: 20 minutes | Cooking Time: 35–38 minutes | Total Time: 55–58 minutes

A good portion of the prep time for this recipe consists of waiting for the tofu to drain. This dish is well worth the wait, especially when spooned over cooked jasmine rice.

2 tablespoons cornstarch

2 tablespoons extra-virgin olive oil, divided

14 ounces extra firm tofu, pressed

1 (7–8 ounce) jar hoisin sauce

2 tablespoons fresh orange juice

1 teaspoon Asian five-spice powder

½ white onion, thinly sliced

½ cup slivered bell pepper

1. Place the cornstarch in a small plastic bag and set aside.

2. Place 1 tablespoon of the oil in another small plastic bag and set aside.

3. Cut the tofu into 1-inch cubes.

4. Place the tofu in the bag of cornstarch and shake to coat thoroughly.

5. Remove the cubes from the cornstarch bag, place them in the oil bag, and shake.

6. Cook the tofu in the air fryer basket at 330°F for 17 to 20 minutes.

7. While the tofu is cooking, prepare the vegetables and place them in the baking pan with the remaining tablespoon of oil.

8. When the tofu has finished, cook the vegetables at 390°F for 5 minutes.

9. Stir the vegetables and cook for 5 more minutes.

10. In a small bowl, mix the hoisin sauce, orange juice, and five-spice powder together.

11. Stir the tofu and hoisin mixture into the baking pan with the vegetables and cook at 390°F for 5 minutes.

12. Gently stir and cook for 3 more minutes.

> **VARIATION:** To press tofu, cover a dinner plate with several layers of paper towel. Put the tofu on the paper towel, cover with several more layers of paper towel, and place another dinner plate on top. Add heavy weight such as a large vegetable can on the plate. Press for at least 30 minues. Drain.

Tofu Sticks with Sweet & Sour Sauce

Yield: 4 servings | Prep Time: 45 minutes | Cooking Time: 6–7 minutes per batch (2 batches) | Total Time: 57–59 minutes

Use the sauce for dipping, as below, or make this recipe into a salad. Simply toss shredded Napa cabbage with orange wedges and sliced almonds, top with the tofu sticks, and drizzle with the sauce for dressing.

2 tablespoons low-sodium soy sauce

1 teaspoon rice vinegar

2 teaspoons sesame oil

14 ounces extra firm tofu, pressed

Sauce

³/₄ cup pineapple juice

1 tablespoon vegan teriyaki sauce

1 tablespoon coconut sugar

¹/₂ teaspoon crushed red pepper flakes

¹/₄ cup water, plus 1 tablespoon

1 tablespoon cornstarch

¹/₂ cup potato starch

¹/₂ cup almond milk

³/₄ cup crushed cornflake crumbs

oil for misting or cooking spray

1. In a shallow container with a lid, mix the soy sauce, vinegar, and oil.

2. Cut the tofu crosswise into sticks, approximately ¹/₂ x ³/₄ x 3¹/₂ inches.

3. Place the tofu sticks in the marinade and refrigerate for 30 minutes.

4. Next make the sauce. In a small saucepan, combine the pineapple juice, teriyaki sauce, sugar, red pepper flakes, and ¹/₄ cup water.

5. Heat the sauce to boiling and then add the cornstarch and the remaining tablespoon of water. Cook just until sauce the thickens and remove from heat.

6. When you're ready to cook the tofu, preheat the air fryer to 390°F.

7. Place the potato starch in one shallow dish, the milk in a second shallow dish, and the cornflake crumbs in a third.

8. Dip the marinated tofu sticks in the starch, then the milk, and then the crumbs.

9. Mist the tofu sticks with oil or cooking spray and place half of them in the air fryer basket in a single layer with space around them.

10. Cook them for 6 to 7 minutes, until crispy. The crust should look dark brown but not burned.

11. Repeat step 10 to cook the remaining tofu sticks.

12. Serve with the sweet & sour sauce for dipping.

Vegetable Turnovers

Yield: 8 turnovers | Prep Time: 15 minutes | Cooking Time: 15 minutes per batch (2 batches) | Total Time: 45 minutes

These are a great dish to take on a picnic. No need to reheat them, though. Just serve them at room temperature.

Vegetable Filling

½ (12-ounce) package frozen California-blend vegetables, thawed

2 tablespoons mirepoix

3 ounces water, plus 1 tablespoon for slurry

1 tablespoon cornstarch

Turnover Crust

1½ cups self-rising flour

2 tablespoons all-vegetable shortening

½ cup almond milk

¼–½ cup all-purpose flour for dusting

oil for misting

NOTE: Mirepoix consists of diced carrots, celery, and onions. Most grocery stores carry it fresh in the vegetable or deli department or frozen. If yours doesn't, you can make your own: ⅓ cup of each ingredient would suffice for this recipe.

1. First make the filling. Coarsely chop the California-blend vegetables.

2. In a small saucepan, cook the vegetables and mirepoix in 3 ounces of water until the vegetables become tender.

3. In a small bowl, stir together the cornstarch with 1 tablespoon of water to make a slurry.

4. Stir the slurry into the vegetable mixture, bring it to a boil, and boil for 2 to 3 minutes, until the sauce thickens.

5. Remove the vegetable filling from the heat and set aside.

6. Next make the crust. In a medium bowl, cut the shortening into the flour until well distributed.

7. Stir in the milk and form the dough into a smooth ball.

8. Dust a clean work surface with 2 tablespoons all-purpose flour.

9. Divide the dough into 2 equal portions.

10. Working with one ball of dough at a time, roll it out to ⅛-inch thickness, keeping it as square as possible.

11. Cut the dough into 4 equal squares.

12. Spoon 1 tablespoon of the filling slightly off center into each dough square.

13. With a finger dipped in water, moisten the edges of each square.

14. Fold one corner over to meet the opposite corner, forming a triangle, and press the edges to seal the turnover.

15. Use a fork to crimp all sides to ensure a tight seal.

16. Spray both sides of the turnovers with oil and cook at 360°F for 15 minutes.

17. Repeat steps 10 through 16 to cook the remaining batch.

VEGETABLES & SIDES

Asparagus Hot Pot

Yield: 4–6 servings | Prep Time: 5 minutes | Cooking Time: 9 minutes | Total Time: 14 minutes

FAST   SUPER EASY

Fresh asparagus is wonderful, but out of season it can cost a lot. Keep a bag or two in your freezer for a quick side dish.

---

2 (10-ounce) bags frozen asparagus

1 tablespoon extra-virgin olive oil

1 tablespoon lemon juice

1 teaspoon vegan Worcestershire sauce

¼ cup grated Parmesan-style topping

1. In a medium bowl, toss the asparagus with the olive oil, lemon juice, and vegan Worcestershire sauce.

2. Pour the asparagus into the air fryer baking pan and cook at 360°F for 7 minutes.

3. Sprinkle with the vegan Parmesan cheese and cook an additional 2 minutes.

Asparagus Roasted

Yield: 4 servings | Prep Time: 5 minutes | Cooking Time: 9–10 minutes | Total Time: 14–15 minutes

FAST GLUTEN FREE SUPER EASY

Our rule of thumb for fresh asparagus is to keep seasonings simple. Omit the tarragon if you like, or substitute other herbs, but whatever you choose, go easy on the herbs and spices to allow the delicate, natural flavor of the vegetable to shine.

1 bunch asparagus (approximately 1 pound)

salt and pepper

1/8 teaspoon dried tarragon, crushed (optional)

1–2 teaspoons extra-light olive oil

1. Wash the asparagus and remove the woody stems.

2. Spread the spears on a cutting board or baking sheet.

3. Sprinkle with salt, pepper, and tarragon or other seasoning.

4. Drizzle 1 teaspoon of oil over the spears and roll them around to coat evenly. If needed, add up to 1 more teaspoon of oil, rolling as you drizzle until all of the spears are coated lightly.

5. Place the spears in the air fryer basket, bending to fit if necessary. They don't have to lie flat.

6. Cook at 390°F for 5 minutes.

7. Shake the basket or stir to redistribute and cook for 4 to 5 more minutes, until they're crisp-tender. Watch the spears closely and don't overcook.

See insert B6 for recipe photo.

TIP: Save the woody stems of the asparagus for making your next batch of veggie broth.

Avocado Boats

Yield: 4 servings | Prep Time: 5 minutes | Cooking Time: 6–8 minutes | Total Time: 11–13 minutes

FAST   GLUTEN FREE   SUPER EASY

Avocados are a nutritious and filling fruit full of healthy omega-3 fatty acids. Served for lunch, these stuffed avocados will help stave off hunger all afternoon.

1 cup frozen white or yellow corn, thawed and drained

1 cup cooked black beans, drained

¼ cup chopped onion

½ teaspoon Tex-Mex Seasoning (page 159)

2 teaspoons lime juice

salt and pepper

2 large avocados

1 (6-ounce) small jar jalapeño slices

Sriracha sauce

1. Mix together the corn, beans, onion, Tex-Mex seasoning, and lime juice. Season to taste with salt and pepper.

2. Halve the avocados and remove the pits.

3. Scoop out some of the flesh in the center of each avocado half, about 1 tablespoon.

4. Divide the corn mixture evenly among the cavities.

5. Place the avocado halves in the air fryer basket and cook at 360°F for 6 to 8 minutes, until the corn mixture is hot.

6. To serve, top with jalapeño slices and pass the Sriracha sauce at the table.

> **NOTE:** Make sure the corn and beans are well drained before mixing.
>
> **TIP:** If we pretend that you're not going to eat that avocado that you scoop out in step 3, put it in a small bowl, mash it with a little lime juice and Tex-Mex Seasoning, and spoon it over the cooked boats before serving.

Barbecue Bellas

Yield: 8 mushrooms | Prep Time: 15 minutes | Cooking Time: 8 minutes | Total Time: 23 minutes

SUPER EASY   TASTER FAVORITE

Fresh pineapple adds a bright, sweet, and fruity taste to plain old bottled barbecue sauce. Choose your favorite brand to make these morsels a must-eat treat.

oil for misting or cooking spray

8 baby bella mushrooms, 2½ inches in diameter

½ cup barbecue sauce

½ cup diced fresh pineapple

1. Spray the air fryer basket with cooking spray or oil.

2. Remove the stems from the mushroom caps and discard or save for alternate use.

3. Use a knife to scrape the dark gills from the underside of the caps.

4. In a small bowl, mix the barbecue sauce and pineapple together.

5. Spoon the barbecue pineapple mixture into the caps.

6. Carefully place the caps into the prepared air fryer basket and cook at 375°F for 8 minutes.

NOTE: If your caps are a bit larger or you want to double the recipe, you can stack them on top of each other to cook in one batch.

TIP: Save the mushroom stems for making your next batch of veggie broth.

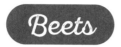

Beets

Yield: 4–8 servings | Prep Time: 5 minutes | Cooking Time: 35–40 minutes | Total Time: 40–45 minutes

GLUTEN FREE **SUPER EASY**

Beets offer a variety of health benefits, and roasting them whole brings out all their natural flavors and sweetness. See the variations below for a few ideas on how versatile they can be.

3 large beets (about 2 pounds)

1. Remove the leaves but leave 1 inch of beet stems intact. Don't cut off the root tails.

2. Wash the beets, pat them dry, and place them in the air fryer basket.

3. Cook at 390°F for approximately 35 to 40 minutes. Cooking time will depend on the size of the beets. (See note below.)

4. When the beets cool enough to handle, cut off the root and stem ends and peel them.

> **NOTE:** The above cooking time works well for 3 large beets with a total weight of approximately 2 pounds. Smaller beets will cook faster, so check for doneness at about 20 minutes—or earlier depending on the size of the vegetables.
>
> **VARIATIONS:** You can enjoy these beets plain, but they also work well in a wide range of dishes. Add chilled, cubed beets to a mixed green salad with vinaigrette or other light dressing. Combine cubed beets with other vegetable chunks to make a hot or cold vegetable salad. Add sliced beets to bean burgers, sandwiches, or even pizza. You can incorporate pureed beets into everything from hummus to brownies.

Broccoli-Rice Casserole

Yield: 8 servings | Prep Time: 15 minutes | Cooking Time: 20 minutes | Total Time: 35 minutes

GLUTEN FREE   SUPER EASY

Broccoli Rice Casserole makes a nice side dish to go along with a Meatless Loaf (page 64).

---

oil for misting or cooking spray

1 (16-ounce) package soft silken tofu

½ cup Cheddar-style shreds

1 teaspoon salt

2 tablespoons almond milk

1 (12-ounce) package chopped broccoli, thawed

1 cup cooked rice

1. Spray the air fryer baking pan with oil or nonstick spray.

2. In a large bowl, beat together the tofu, cheese shreds, salt, and milk with an electric mixer until they combine.

3. Stir in the broccoli and rice.

4. Spoon the casserole mixture into the prepared baking pan.

5. Cook at 360°F for 20 minutes.

Brussels Sprouts

Yield: 3 servings | Prep Time: 5 minutes | Cooking Time: 5 minutes | Total Time: 10 minutes

FAST   GLUTEN FREE   SUPER EASY

Fresh Brussels sprouts taste great, but some people don't love the powerful aroma that they can produce. The secret is to use frozen sprouts. You'll avoid the complaints and save time too.

---

1 (10-ounce) package frozen Brussels sprouts, thawed

2 teaspoons olive oil

1 teaspoon maple syrup

salt and pepper

2 tablespoons chopped walnuts

1. Cut the sprouts in half lengthwise.

2. In a small bowl, mix together the oil and syrup.

3. Pour the oil mixture over the sprout halves and toss to mix well.

4. Place the sprouts in the air fryer basket and season to taste with salt and pepper.

5. Cook at 360°F for approximately 5 minutes, until the edges begin to brown.

6. Transfer the sprouts to a serving dish, top them with the walnuts, and serve hot.

Butternut Squash

Yield: 4 servings | Prep Time: 15 minutes | Cooking Time: 8–9 minutes | Total Time: 23–24 minutes

GLUTEN FREE

The aromatic spices in this recipe may remind you of fall, but you should enjoy this slightly sweet side dish any time you can find butternut squash at your local grocery store—which is usually year-round!

Squash

1 butternut squash (about 2 pounds)

$^1/_4$ teaspoon salt

$^1/_4$ teaspoon cinnamon

1 tablespoon olive oil

Sauce

2 tablespoons vegan butter

2 tablespoons maple syrup

$^1/_4$ teaspoon salt

$^1/_4$ teaspoon ground ginger

$^1/_4$ teaspoon cinnamon

1. Peel the squash, remove the seeds, and cut it into $^1/_2$-inch cubes.

2. In a large bowl, add the squash cubes, sprinkle them with seasonings, and stir to coat thoroughly.

3. Drizzle the olive oil over the squash cubes and stir again to coat evenly.

4. Place the squash in the air fryer basket and cook at 390°F for 4 minutes.

5. Shake the basket and cook for 4 to 5 more minutes or just until tender. Then transfer to a serving bowl.

6. Place all of the sauce ingredients in the air fryer baking pan and cook at 390°F for 30 seconds or long enough to melt the vegan butter and heat the other ingredients.

7. Stir the sauce to blend the ingredients and pour it over the squash.

8. Stir the squash cubes and sauce together to coat evenly.

Carrot Pudding

Yield: 4 servings | Prep Time: 20-22 minutes | Cooking Time: 30 minutes | Total Time: 50–52 minutes

Carrot Pudding is a delicious side with the Meatless Loaf (page 64) or Brown Rice Bake (page 54). Leftovers can be reheated for breakfast.

2 (12-ounce) bags frozen sliced carrots, partially thawed

½ cup water

cooking spray

2 tablespoons Bob's Red Mill egg replacer

4 tablespoons plant-based milk

¼ cup maple syrup

1½ teaspoons baking powder

1½ teaspoons vanilla

1 teaspoon cinnamon

1 teaspoon nutmeg

2 tablespoons all-purpose flour

1. Coarsely chop the carrots and place them in a medium-size cooking pot with the water.

2. On high heat, bring the water and carrots to a boil.

3. Reduce the heat to medium and cook for 8 to 10 minutes until tender.

4. Spray a baking pan with nonstick spray and set aside.

5. Drain the carrots and puree in a food processor.

6. Transfer to a medium-size bowl.

7. In a small bowl, mix the egg replacer and plant-based milk together.

8. Pour the mixture into the carrots and add the remaining ingredients.

9. Using an electric mixer, beat the mixture until smooth.

10. Pour the mixture into a baking pan.

11. Cook at 360°F for 30 minutes.

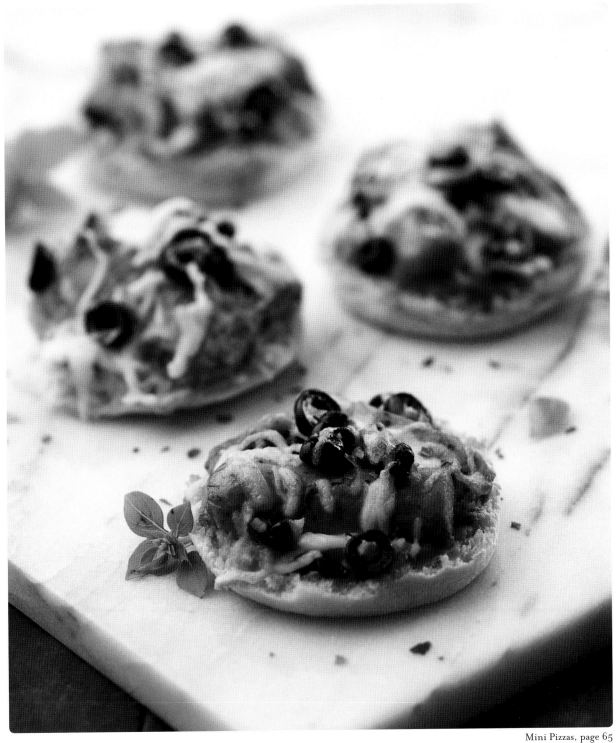

Mini Pizzas, page 65

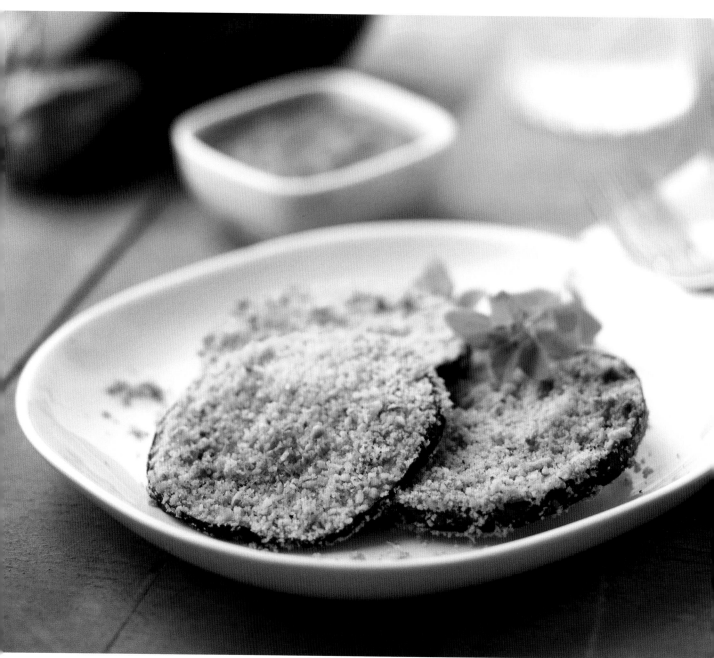

Pecan-Crusted Eggplant, page 67

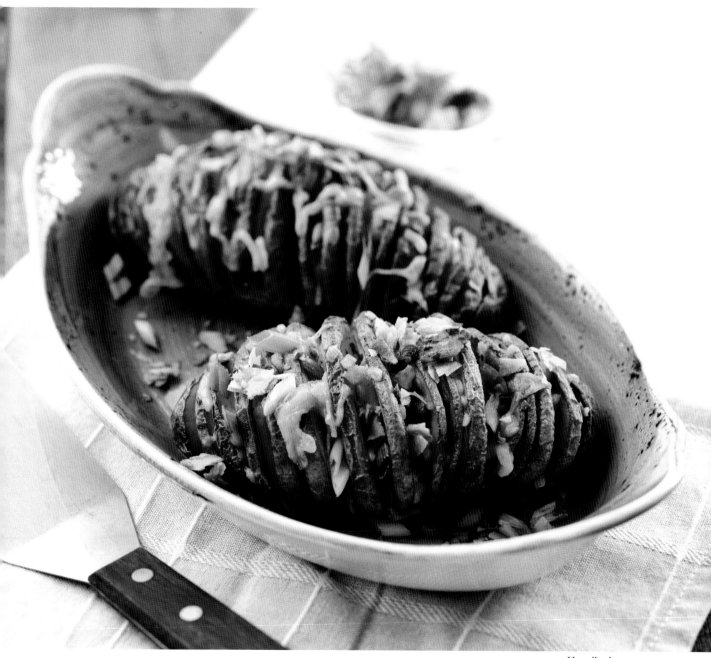

Hasselbacks, page 93

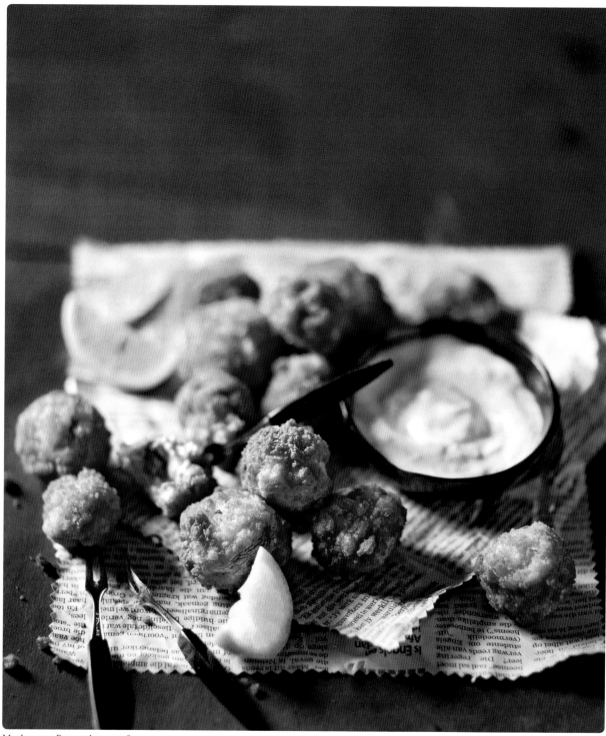

Mushrooms Battered, page 96

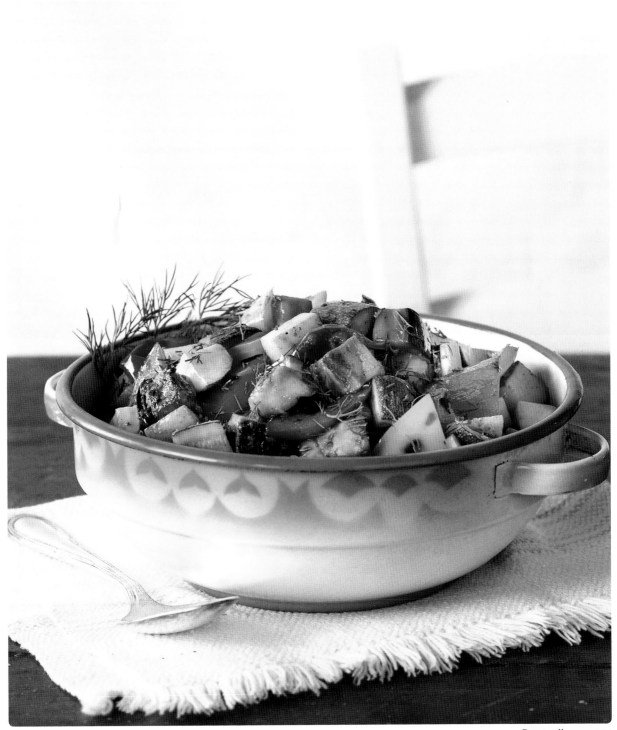

Ratatouille, page 105

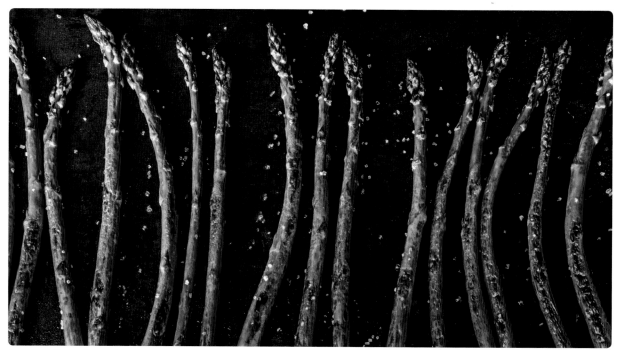

Asparagus Roasted, page 79

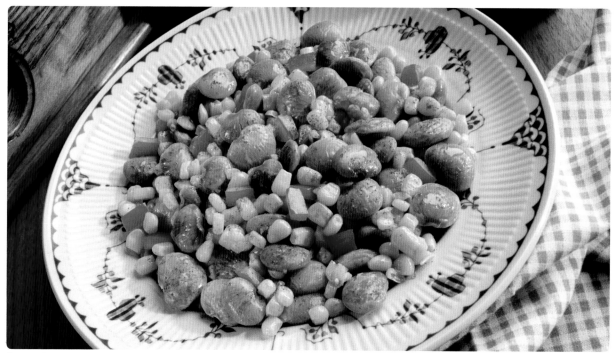

Succotash, page 109

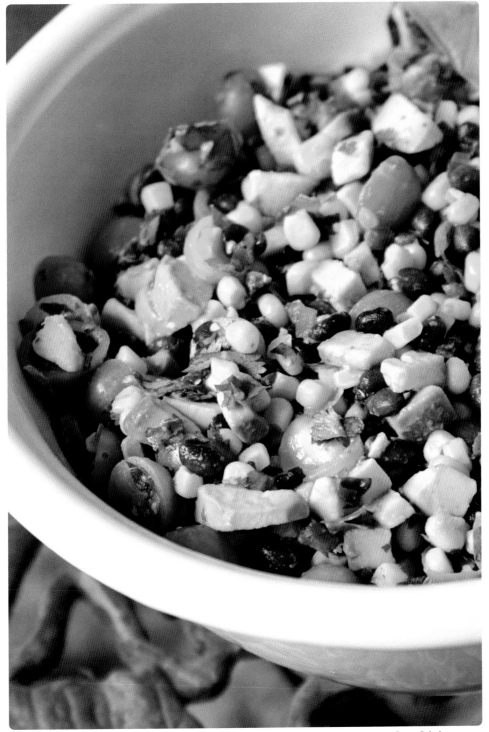

Corn Salad, page 115

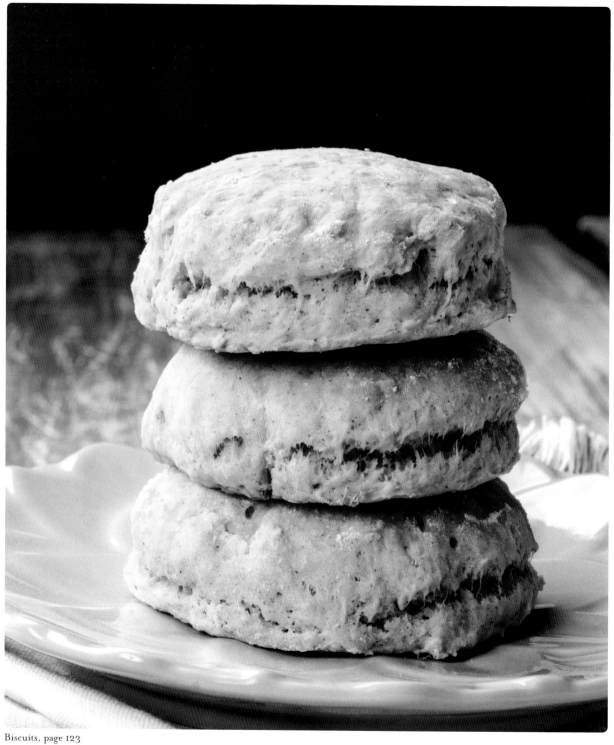

Biscuits, page 123

Carrots Glazed

Yield: 4 servings | Prep Time: 10 minutes | Cooking Time: 8–10 minutes | Total Time: 18–20 minutes

GLUTEN FREE   KID FRIENDLY   SUPER EASY

The glaze in this recipe adds a nice flavor that transforms the carrots into a more interesting side dish. If you prefer the natural taste of roasted carrots just as they are, and you don't need to sweeten the deal, simply omit the glaze below.

---

2 teaspoons pure maple syrup

1 teaspoon orange juice

$\frac{1}{2}$ teaspoon grated orange rind

$\frac{1}{8}$ teaspoon ginger

1 pound peeled baby carrots

2 teaspoons olive oil

$\frac{1}{4}$ teaspoon salt

1. In a small bowl, combine the maple syrup, orange juice, grated rind, and ginger and set aside.

2. Toss the carrots with the oil and salt to coat well.

3. Cook at 390°F for 5 minutes.

4. Shake the basket to redistribute the carrots and cook for 2 to 4 more minutes, until they are barely tender.

5. Transfer the carrots to the air fryer baking pan.

6. Stir the syrup mixture again, pour it over the carrots, and stir to coat.

7. Cook at 360°F until heated through, about 1 minute.

Coconut-Curry Pineapple

Yield: 8 servings | Prep Time: 15 minutes | Cooking Time: 20 minutes | Total Time: 35 minutes

GLUTEN FREE   SUPER EASY

The curry gives this simple dish a burst of amazing flavor. Serve it as a side garnished with a few green onion slices, pour it over cooked jasmine or basmati rice, or spoon it over nondairy frozen dessert for a delicious after-dinner snack. It's that versatile!

3¾ cups fresh pineapple

oil for misting or cooking spray

1 cup unsweetened coconut flakes

1 teaspoon curry powder

1½ cups coconut milk

1. Dice the pineapple into ⅛-inch chunks.

2. Spray the air fryer baking pan with oil or cooking spray.

3. In a large bowl, mix the pineapple chunks, coconut flakes, and curry powder.

4. Spoon the pineapple mixture into the air fryer baking pan and pour the coconut milk over it.

5. Cook at 360°F for 20 minutes.

Corn Croquettes

Yield: 4 servings | Prep Time: 10 minutes | Cooking Time: 15–18 minutes | Total Time: 22–24 minutes

SUPER EASY   **TASTER FAVORITE**

These croquettes work best with slightly firm mashed potatoes. If your leftovers seem too moist, try adding a little potato starch or plain breadcrumbs to absorb some of the liquid and thicken the potatoes. Also make sure to drain the corn well.

¼ cup chopped red bell pepper

¼ cup chopped poblano pepper

oil for misting

½ cup leftover mashed potatoes

1½ cups frozen corn kernels, thawed and drained

½ teaspoon onion powder

¼ teaspoon ground cumin

⅛ teaspoon ground black pepper

¼ teaspoon salt

½ cup panko breadcrumbs

1. Place the chopped peppers in the air fryer baking pan and mist with oil.

2. Cook at 390°F for 3 to 4 minutes to soften them slightly.

3. Meanwhile, in a medium bowl, stir together the potatoes, corn, and seasonings.

4. Add the cooked peppers to the potato mixture and stir thoroughly.

5. Shape the veggie mixture into 16 balls.

6. Roll the balls in the breadcrumbs, mist them with oil, and place them in the air fryer basket.

7. Cook at 360°F for 12 to 14 minutes, until the croquettes turn golden brown and crispy.

VARIATION: Some like it hot! For super-spicy croquettes, substitute fresh jalapeños for the poblano peppers.

Fingerling Potatoes

Yield: 4 servings | Prep Time: 5 minutes | Cooking Time: 12–18 minutes | Total Time: 17–23 minutes

FAST   GLUTEN FREE   GREAT SNACK   SUPER EASY

Nutritional yeast gives these potatoes a nice boost in flavor and some extra protein too. Serve them for breakfast, lunch, or dinner as a hearty and filling accompaniment to your meal.

1 pound fingerling potatoes

2 tablespoons nutritional yeast

2 teaspoons lemon pepper seasoning

2 tablespoons light olive oil

salt

1. Cut the potatoes in half lengthwise.

2. In a large bowl, combine the potatoes, yeast, and lemon pepper. Stir to distribute the seasonings evenly.

3. Add the oil and stir well to coat the potatoes thoroughly.

4. Place the potatoes in the air fryer basket and cook at 390°F for 12 to 18 minutes, until they lightly brown and are tender inside.

5. Taste and, if needed, sprinkle with salt before serving.

French Fries

Yield: 4 servings | Prep Time: 10 minutes | Cooking Time: 25 minutes | Total Time: 35 minutes

GLUTEN FREE GREAT SNACK KID FRIENDLY SUPER EASY

We Americans love our French fries! Thanks to the air fryer, we can enjoy the great taste without all the guilt.

---

2 cups fresh potatoes

2 teaspoons light olive oil

½ teaspoon salt

1. Cut the potatoes into ½-inch slices.
2. Cut each slice into ½-inch fries.
3. Rinse the raw fries and blot them dry with a clean towel.
4. Place the fries, oil, and salt in a plastic bag or a container with lid. Shake to mix them well and coat evenly.
5. Pile the fries in the air fryer basket.
6. Cook at 390°F for 10 minutes.
7. Shake the basket to redistribute fries and continue cooking for about 15 minutes or until the fries turn golden brown.

Green Beans Sesame

Yield: 4 servings | Prep Time: 10 minutes | Cooking Time: 17–22 minutes | Total Time: 27–32 minutes

Crushed red pepper flakes give these beans a little kick, but they're optional. The other seasonings stand alone quite well, so, for picky eaters or sensitive palates, you can omit the red pepper and still have a tasty, flavorful dish.

1 pound fresh green beans

1 tablespoon sesame oil

½ medium onion, julienned

1 tablespoon sesame seeds

¼ teaspoon crushed red pepper flakes

oil for misting

1 tablespoon soy sauce

1. Wash the beans and snap off the stem ends.

2. In a large bowl, toss the beans with the sesame oil.

3. Place them in the air fryer basket and cook at 330°F for 5 minutes.

4. Shake the basket and cook for 5 more minutes.

5. If needed, continue cooking for 2 to 4 minutes, until the beans are as tender as you like. They may shrivel slightly and brown in places.

6. Remove from the basket and set aside.

7. Place the slivered onion in the air fryer baking pan. Stir in the sesame seeds and red pepper and mist with oil.

8. Cook for 5 minutes.

9. Stir and, if needed, cook 2 to 3 more minutes until the onion becomes crisp-tender.

10. Stir the soy sauce into the onions. Pour the onion mixture over the green beans and stir well to combine.

TIP: If you get to step 10 and the beans have cooled too much, do a quick reheat. Toss them back into the air fryer basket, cook at 390°F for 1 or 2 minutes, then combine them with the onion mixture.

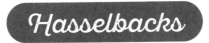
Hasselbacks

Yield: 4 servings | Prep Time: 10 minutes | Cooking Time: 41 minutes | Total Time: 51 minutes

GLUTEN FREE **TASTER FAVORITE**

This familiar favorite is often served as a side, but it also makes a terrific lunch when you want something that will stick to your ribs. Add a side salad and you have a healthy, balanced meal with staying power.

2 large potatoes, about 1 pound each

oil for misting or cooking spray

salt and pepper

garlic powder

1½ ounces Cheddar-style shreds

¼ cup chopped green onion tops

vegan sour cream (optional)

Coconut Bacon (page 3) (optional)

1. Preheat the air fryer to 390°F.

2. Scrub the potatoes and slice them crosswise every ¼ to ½ inch about ¾ of the way through. You want the bottom of the potato to remain intact.

3. Fan the potatoes slightly to separate the slices and mist them with oil.

4. Sprinkle the slices to taste with salt, pepper, and garlic powder. The uncooked potatoes won't bend easily, so press a little of the oil and seasonings down between the slices.

5. Place the potatoes in the air fryer basket and cook for 40 minutes or until the centers test done when pierced with a fork.

6. Top the potatoes with cheese shreds, pushing some down between the slices.

7. Cook 30 to 60 more seconds to melt the cheese.

8. Cut each potato in half crosswise, sprinkle with the green onions, and serve hot.

9. Top with vegan sour cream and Coconut Bacon if you like.

See insert B3 for recipe photo.

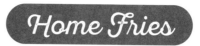

Home Fries

Yield: 3–4 servings | Prep Time: 8 minutes | Cooking Time: 20–25 minutes | Total Time: 28–33 minutes

GLUTEN FREE   KID FRIENDLY   SUPER EASY

Home fries taste great with any meal. Serve them plain, seasoned, sprinkled with vegan cheese shreds, or topped with your favorite condiments. Any way you try them, they're fantastic.

3 pounds potatoes

½ teaspoon oil

salt and pepper

1. Cut the potatoes into 1-inch cubes.

2. In a large bowl, add the potatoes and oil and stir to coat thoroughly.

3. Pour the potatoes into the air fryer basket and cook at 390°F for 10 minutes.

4. Shake the basket to redistribute the home fries and continue cooking for about 10 to 15 minutes or until the potatoes turn brown and crisp.

5. Season with salt and pepper to taste.

VARIATIONS: In step 2, add ½ teaspoon of onion powder for a little extra zing. Experiment with garlic powder or other spices and really make this recipe your own. Also see the Sweet Potato Home Fries recipe on page 110.

Mushroom Sauté

Yield: 2–4 servings | Prep Time: 5 minutes | Cooking Time: 4–5 minutes | Total Time: 9–10 minutes

FAST SUPER EASY

This is almost too simple to qualify as a recipe, but we didn't want to omit such a handy reference. For any other type of mushroom, you may need to adjust the cooking time slightly.

8 ounces sliced white mushrooms

¼ teaspoon garlic powder

1 tablespoon vegan Worcestershire sauce

1. Rinse and drain the mushrooms well.

2. In a large bowl, add the mushrooms and sprinkle them with the garlic powder and vegan Worcestershire sauce. Stir well to distribute evenly.

3. Place the mushrooms in the air fryer basket and cook at 390°F for 4 to 5 minutes, until the mushrooms become tender.

Mushrooms Battered

Yield: 4 servings | Prep Time: 10 minutes | Cooking Time: 10–12 minutes | Total Time: 20–22 minutes

GREAT SNACK   TASTER FAVORITE

Many foods with a high moisture content can prove challenging to cook in an air fryer. Mushrooms are definitely an exception. The coating in this recipe contains panko for maximum crunch, and these actually taste *better* than the deep-fried version.

1 tablespoon Bob's Red Mill egg replacer

2 tablespoons water

8 ounces whole white button mushrooms

1/2 teaspoon salt

1/8 teaspoon pepper

1/4 teaspoon garlic powder

5 tablespoons potato starch

2 tablespoons almond milk

1 cup panko breadcrumbs

oil for misting or cooking spray

1. In a small bowl, whisk the egg replacer and water together and set aside to thicken.

2. Place the breadcrumbs on a plate or in a shallow dish.

3. In a large bowl, add the mushrooms, salt, pepper, and garlic powder and stir well to distribute the seasonings evenly.

4. Add the potato starch to the mushrooms and toss to coat well.

5. Add the almond milk to the egg mixture and whisk to combine well.

6. Dip the mushrooms in the milk mixture, then roll them in the breadcrumbs.

7. Mist the breaded mushrooms with oil and place them in the air fryer basket. It's fine if you have to crowd them, and you may have to stack a few.

8. Cook at 390°F for 5 minutes.

9. Shake the basket to rearrange the mushrooms. If you see any white spots, mist them with oil. Cook for 5 to 7 more minutes or until the mushrooms turn golden brown and crispy.

See insert B4 for recipe photo.

Mushrooms in Soy

Yield: 2–4 servings | Prep Time: 5 minutes | Cooking Time: 4–5 minutes | Total Time: 9–10 minutes

FAST   SUPER EASY

This dish tastes great as a simple side dish, and it makes a nice topping for plain brown rice. Pair it with a variety of Asian-inspired dishes.

8 ounces sliced white mushrooms

¼ teaspoon dried rosemary

¼ teaspoon dried thyme

1 tablespoon soy sauce

1. Rinse and drain the mushrooms and place them in a large bowl.

2. Sprinkle the mushrooms with rosemary, thyme, and soy sauce. Stir well to distribute seasonings evenly.

3. Place the mushrooms in the air fryer basket and cook at 390°F for 4 to 5 minutes, until tender.

TIP: You can double this recipe and still cook the mushrooms in one batch. The cooking time will be slightly longer, and you'll need to stop midway and shake to redistribute the mushrooms.

Mushrooms Stuffed

Yield: 4–6 servings | Prep Time: 30 minutes | Cooking Time: 10 minutes | Total Time: 40 minutes

The stuffing below tastes very spicy. If it's too hot for your palate, reduce or eliminate the red pepper flakes.

8 ounces small baby bella mushrooms

1 cup panko breadcrumbs

1 teaspoon red pepper flakes

1 teaspoon ground allspice

1 teaspoon thyme

2 tablespoons grated Parmesan-style topping

4 tablespoons extra-virgin olive oil

oil for misting

1. Remove the stems from the mushrooms, mince the stems, and set them aside in a medium bowl.

2. Using the tip of a knife, scrape the dark gills from the underside of the mushroom caps.

3. Lay the caps on a sheet of wax paper, gill side down.

4. To the bowl of minced stems, add the breadcrumbs, red pepper flakes, allspice, thyme, Parmesan-style topping, and olive oil and mix well.

5. Mist the caps with oil and turn them over, gill side up.

6. Shape the filling into the same number of balls as you have mushroom caps.

7. Press the balls into the caps and place the stuffed caps in the air fryer basket. You should be able to fit them in a single layer if you place them close together. If not, you can stack them.

8. Cook at 360°F for 10 minutes to heat through.

> **NOTE:** We tested this recipe using mushrooms about 2 inches in diameter. Larger mushrooms may take longer to cook through.
>
> **TIP:** The easiest way to mix this stuffing is with your hands. Get out those food-grade gloves and dig in!
>
> **VARIATION:** For a slightly creamier taste, you can substitute melted vegan butter for the olive oil.

Okra & Tomatoes

Yield: 3–4 servings | Prep Time: 10 minutes | Cooking Time: 20–25 minutes | Total Time: 30–35 minutes

GLUTEN FREE   SUPER EASY

Okra & Tomatoes is a staple of our summer suppers.

1 pound fresh okra

1 (15-ounce) can stewed tomatoes

¼ cup mirepoix

1. Trim stem ends off okra and discard or reserve for alternate use.
2. Cut the okra pods into ¼-inch slices and place them in the air fryer baking pan.
3. Sprinkle the mirepoix over the okra.
4. Pour the stewed tomatoes, including the juice, over the okra as well.
5. Cook at 390°F for 20 to 25 minutes, until the okra becomes tender.

NOTE: Frozen mirepoix is such a great standby that it's a staple in both of our kitchens. If you can't find it frozen or premade, you can make it fresh quite easily. Dice up equal amounts of onions, celery, and carrots.

TIP: Save the okra stems for making your next batch of veggie broth.

Okra Battered

Yield: 4 servings | Prep Time: 15 minutes | Cooking Time: 12–15 minutes | Total Time: 27–30 minutes

TASTER FAVORITE

If you love breaded, deep-fried okra, you're in for a pleasant surprise. Air frying makes it healthier of course, but this version tastes much better too!

---

1 tablespoon Bob's Red Mill egg replacer

1 cup almond milk

7–8 ounces fresh okra

1 cup plain breadcrumbs

½ teaspoon salt

oil for misting or cooking spray

1. In a large bowl, whisk together the egg replacer and milk and set aside.

2. Remove the stem ends from the okra and discard or reserve for alternate use.

3. Cut the okra pods crosswise into ½-inch slices.

4. Add the okra slices to the milk mixture and stir to coat.

5. In a plastic bag or a container with lid, mix together the breadcrumbs and salt.

6. Using a slotted spoon, remove the okra from the egg mixture, letting the excess drip off, and transfer the slices into the bag or container with breadcrumbs. Remove only a few slices of okra at a time to allow plenty of egg wash to drip off. Drain the okra well before you place it in the breadcrumbs.

7. Shake the okra in the crumbs to coat well.

8. Place all of the coated okra into the air fryer basket and mist with oil or cooking spray. The okra doesn't have to fit in a single later, and you don't need to spray all sides at this point. A good spritz on top will do.

9. Cook at 390°F for 5 minutes.

10. Shake the basket to rearrange the okra and spritz with oil as you shake.

11. Cook 5 more minutes.

12. Shake and spray again, covering any white spots you may have missed.

13. Cook for 2 to 5 more minutes or until the okra turns golden brown and crispy.

> **TIP:** Save the okra stems for making your next batch of veggie broth.
>
> **VARIATION:** For an extra-crispy version, substitute panko for half (or all) of the plain breadcrumbs.

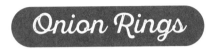

Onion Rings

Yield: 4 servings | Prep Time: 15 minutes | Cooking Time: 12–14 minutes | Total Time: 27–29 minutes

GREAT SNACK   TASTER FAVORITE

Onion rings deep-fried in oil soak up loads of grease. This version is healthier and tastes a whole lot better too!

---

1 large onion (see Tip below)

½ cup all-purpose white flour, plus 2 tablespoons

½ teaspoon salt

½ cup beer, plus 2 tablespoons

1 cup crushed panko breadcrumbs

oil for misting or cooking spray

1. Slice the onion crosswise and separate it into rings.

2. In a large bowl, mix together the flour and salt.

3. Slowly pour the beer into the flour mixture. Stir until it stops foaming and turns into a thick batter.

4. Place the onion rings in the batter and stir to coat them well.

5. Place the breadcrumbs in a plastic bag or a container with a lid.

6. Working with a few at a time, remove the onion rings from the batter, shake off the excess, and drop them into the breadcrumbs. Shake the bag or container to coat the onions, then lay them out on a baking sheet or wax paper.

7. When you've breaded all of the rings, spray both sides with oil and pile them into the air fryer basket.

8. Cook at 390°F for 5 minutes.

9. Shake the basket, mist the rings with oil again, and cook for 5 more minutes.

10. Mist again and cook for an additional 2 to 4 minutes, until the rings turn golden brown and crispy.

NOTE: You can't stack a lot of foods in air fryers because multiple layers pack down and block air flow, which is of course a vital part of the cooking process. Onion rings are different. Stacking is fine because, even if they overlap, plenty of air can circulate through all of the gaps.

TIP: We recommend a 1015 or Vidalia onion for this recipe.

Peas with Mint & Lemon

Yield: 4 servings | Prep Time: 5 minutes | Cooking Time: 5 minutes | Total Time: 10 minutes

FAST   GLUTEN FREE   SUPER EASY

These delicately cooked green peas are super fast and crazy easy, and the brilliant color will perk up any meal. Serve them à la carte or toss them into salads, sides, or main dishes.

1 (10-ounce) package frozen green peas, thawed

½ teaspoon grated lemon zest

1 tablespoon fresh mint, shredded (optional)

1 teaspoon melted vegan butter

1. Toss together the peas, lemon zest, mint (if using), and melted butter.

2. Place the peas in the air fryer basket and cook at 360°F for approximately 5 minutes, until the peas are nice and hot.

Peas with Mushrooms & Tarragon

Yield: 4 servings | Prep Time: 15 minutes | Cooking Time: 10 minutes | Total Time: 25 minutes

GLUTEN FREE **SUPER EASY**

Our local market rarely sells fresh green peas, but you definitely should use them if your grocery store carries them. Frozen are nearly as good and make a great substitute for this recipe.

½ cup vegetable broth

2½ cups fresh green peas

1 cup finely diced mushrooms

½ cup thinly sliced green onions

1½ teaspoons dried tarragon

½ teaspoon salt

1. In a medium bowl, add the peas, mushrooms, onions, tarragon, and salt to the vegetable broth and stir.

2. Pour the mushroom mixture into the air fryer baking pan.

3. Cook at 360°F for 5 minutes.

4. Stir and cook for 5 more minutes.

VARIATION: If you can't find fresh peas, use 1 (12-ounce) package of frozen peas and thaw them before cooking.

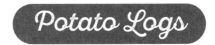

Potato Logs

Yield: 3–4 servings | Prep Time: 5 minutes | Cooking Time: 10–15 minutes | Total Time: 15–20 minutes

FAST   SUPER EASY   TASTER FAVORITE

If you love thick-cut fries, you can make a meal of these potato logs. For a nice bright and tangy complement to the earthy vegan Parmesan, try dipping them in marinara sauce.

1 pound medium Yukon Gold potatoes

¾ cup dry plain breadcrumbs

¼ cup grated Parmesan-style topping

½ teaspoon garlic powder

½ teaspoon salt

oil for misting or cooking spray

1. Cut the potatoes lengthwise into thick wedges, placing them in a bowl of water as you go to prevent browning.

2. In a shallow dish, mix together the breadcrumbs, Parmesan topping, garlic powder, and salt.

3. Working with a few at a time, remove the potatoes from the water—without drying them—and roll them in the breadcrumb mixture.

4. Spray the air fryer basket with cooking spray and add the potato logs. The potatoes don't have to fit in a single layer.

5. Cook at 390°F for 8 minutes.

6. Shake the basket and cook for 2 to 7 more minutes, until the coating is crisp and the potatoes are done inside.

> **NOTE:** Total cooking time can vary greatly depending on the size of your potatoes, the thickness of the wedges, and how crowded your air fryer basket may be. If you're using small potatoes or smaller wedges, check early and often in step 6 to prevent burning.

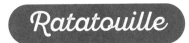

Ratatouille

Yield: 2–3 servings | Prep Time: 20 minutes | Cooking Time: 20 minutes | Total Time: 40 minutes

GLUTEN FREE SUPER EASY

This versatile dish works great as a light lunch or a side dish. The tomatoes burst and mix with the oil to make a lovely sauce.

1½ cups diced zucchini (½-inch dice)

1½ cups diced yellow crookneck squash (½-inch dice)

½ cup diced bell peppers (½-inch dice)

½ cup diced onion (½-inch dice)

1–3 cloves garlic, minced

1 tablespoon extra-virgin olive oil

1 tablespoon Tuscan Herb Mix (page 161)

½ teaspoon salt

6–8 cherry tomatoes

1. Combine the zucchini, squash, bell pepper, onion, and garlic with the oil, Tuscan Herb Mix, and salt and toss to coat thoroughly.

2. Spoon the veggie mixture into the air fryer baking pan.

3. Cook at 390°F for 10 minutes.

4. Stir and add the cherry tomatoes.

5. Cook for 10 more minutes and stir before serving.

See insert B5 for recipe photo.

> **TIP:** You want a total of 4 cups of vegetables, excluding the tomatoes, before cooking, so make sure to dice all of the vegetables uniformly.

Root Vegetables

Yield: 3–4 servings | Prep Time: 10 minutes | Cooking Time: 15–20 minutes | Total Time: 25–30 minutes

GLUTEN FREE **SUPER EASY**

This simple yet hearty side dish comes together quickly. Red onions are particularly tasty with potatoes, but you can use whatever you have on hand.

---

2 tablespoons vegetable broth

2 cups small red potatoes

2 cups baby carrots

2 cloves garlic

1 cup slivered onion

1 tablespoon light olive oil

1. Quarter the potatoes, split the carrots lengthwise, and mince the garlic.

2. In a medium bowl, add all ingredients to the vegetable broth and stir to coat evenly.

3. Pour the vegetables into the air fryer basket and cook at 360°F for 15 to 20 minutes, until the vegetables become tender.

Squash Casserole

Yield: 4 servings | Prep Time: 20 minutes | Cooking Time: 35 minutes | Total Time: 55 minutes

TASTER FAVORITE

This tasty side dish is especially delicious when yellow squash are in season. Our test panel raved over this recipe and asked for seconds.

2 cups sliced yellow crookneck squash, ¼-inch thick

1 tablespoon diced bell pepper

1 tablespoon minced onion

2 tablespoons chopped ripe black olives

½ cup Cheddar-style shreds

1 cup panko breadcrumbs

½ teaspoon salt

¼ teaspoon dried thyme

1 teaspoon dried parsley

1 tablespoon minced celery

4 tablespoons vegan butter, melted

oil for misting or cooking spray

1. In a medium saucepan of boiling water, cook the squash slices for 15 minutes, until tender.

2. Drain the slices well and place them in a medium bowl.

3. Add the bell pepper, onion, olives, cheese shreds, breadcrumbs, salt, thyme, parsley, and celery and stir to mix thoroughly.

4. Stir in the vegan butter and mix well until everything is moist and well blended.

5. Spray the air fryer baking pan with oil or cooking spray and pour the casserole mixture into it, pressing it down to make a smooth top.

6. Cook at 360°F for 20 minutes. The top should be lightly browned when done.

TIP: The easiest way to mix the casserole is with your hands. Keep disposable food-grade gloves in your kitchen for messy jobs like this one.

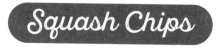

Squash Chips

Yield: 4 servings | Prep Time: 20 minutes | Cooking Time: 10–12 minutes | Total Time: 30–32 minutes

TASTER FAVORITE

Yellow crookneck is one of the most popular squash varieties in the South. We use it in everything from a simple sauté to veggie dressing, but it's hard to beat plain fried squash. This healthier air-fryer version takes a little time but is well worth it.

½ cup almond milk

1½ teaspoons lemon juice

2 tablespoons Bob's Red Mill egg replacer

4 tablespoons water

2 large yellow squash (about ¾ pound)

1 cup panko breadcrumbs, divided

¼ cup white cornmeal

½ teaspoon salt

oil for misting or cooking spray

black pepper

1. In a medium bowl, mix the almond milk and lemon juice.

2. In a small cup, stir together the egg replacer and water.

3. Cut the squash crosswise into ¼-inch-thick rounds.

4. Preheat the air fryer to 390°F.

5. In a plastic bag or a container with a lid, combine ¼ cup of the breadcrumbs, the cornmeal, and salt. Shake to mix well.

6. Place the rest of the breadcrumbs in a shallow dish.

7. Add the egg mixture to the bowl with the almond milk and whisk together.

8. Place all of the squash slices in the almond milk mixture and stir to coat.

9. Lift the squash slices from the liquid using a slotted spoon, letting the excess drip off, and transfer them to the panko-cornmeal mixture. Close the bag or container and shake well to coat.

10. Remove the squash slices from the crumb mixture, again letting the excess fall off. Return the slices to the almond milk mixture and stir gently to coat. If you need more liquid, add a little more almond milk.

11. Taking a few at a time, remove the squash slices from the liquid and dip them into the breadcrumbs in the shallow dish.

12. Spray the squash chips with oil or cooking spray and place them in the air fryer basket. Try to position them in a single layer, but it's OK if the chips crowd and overlap in places.

13. Cook at 390°F for 5 minutes.

14. Shake the basket or use a fork to break up any that have stuck together.

15. Mist again with oil, cook for 5 more minutes, and check the slices again.

16. If necessary, mist again with oil and cook 1 or 2 more minutes until the squash chips are crispy and golden brown.

17. Sprinkle liberally with freshly ground black pepper.

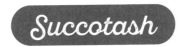

Succotash

Yield: 6–8 servings | Prep Time: 20 minutes | Cooking Time: 15 minutes | Total Time: 35 minutes

GLUTEN FREE   SUPER EASY

Native Americans taught the Pilgrims to cook succotash with fresh ingredients. Frozen lima beans or butterbeans speed up the process considerably.

3 ears corn

1 (12-ounce) package frozen lima beans or butterbeans

½ teaspoon garlic powder

½ cup minced onion

½ cup almond milk

oil for misting or cooking spray

1. Shuck the corn and cut the kernels from the cob. You should have about 3 cups of kernels.

2. In a medium bowl, mix all of the ingredients together.

3. Spray the air fryer baking pan with oil or cooking spray and pour the succotash into it.

4. Cook at 360°F for 10 minutes.

5. Stir and cook for 5 more minutes.

See insert B6 for recipe photo.

Sweet Potato Home Fries

Yield: 4 servings | Prep Time: 10 minutes | Cooking Time: 9–10 minutes | Total Time: 19–20 minutes

GLUTEN FREE   GREAT SNACK   SUPER EASY

This standard side dish pairs well with lots of main courses, but don't forget brunch! Serve this alongside a nice tofu scramble for a late breakfast on a lazy Saturday or Sunday.

2 large sweet potatoes

1 teaspoon garlic powder

½ teaspoon smoked paprika

1 tablespoon light olive oil

oil for misting

salt and pepper

1. Peel and cut the potatoes into ¾-inch cubes (peeling is optional). You should have about 3 cups of cubes.

2. In a large bowl, add the potatoes, sprinkle them with garlic and paprika, and stir well.

3. Drizzle the oil over the potatoes and stir to coat evenly.

4. Place the potatoes in the air fryer basket and cook for 5 minutes at 390°F.

5. Shake the basket or use a spoon to rearrange the potatoes.

6. Mist them with oil and cook for 4 or 5 more minutes, just until tender.

7. Sprinkle the home fries with salt and pepper to taste.

TIP: Take care not to overcook these. Pause during the second cooking time to check for doneness.

Vegetable Couscous

Yield: 4 servings | Prep Time: 15 minutes | Cooking Time: 10–12 minutes | Total Time: 25–27 minutes

This quick and easy dish is filling without being heavy. It pairs well with simple accompaniments, such as fresh sliced tomatoes or sautéed vegetables.

4 ounces fresh white mushrooms

1/2 medium green bell pepper

1 stalk celery

1 cup roughly chopped asparagus

1/4 small onion

1/4 teaspoon ground coriander

1/4 teaspoon ground cumin

salt and pepper

1 tablespoon light olive oil

Couscous

1 cup vegetable broth

3/4 cup uncooked couscous

1/2 teaspoon salt (omit if using salty vegetable broth)

1. Slice the mushrooms, julienne the bell pepper, slice the celery thinly, prepare the asparagus, and sliver the onion.

2. In a large bowl, combine all of the vegetables. Add the coriander, cumin, and salt and pepper to taste and stir to mix well.

3. Add the olive oil and stir again to coat the vegetables evenly.

4. Place the vegetables in the air fryer basket and cook at 390°F for 5 minutes.

5. Stir the veggies and cook for 5 to 7 more minutes, until tender.

6. Meanwhile, in a large saucepan, heat the broth to boiling.

7. Stir the couscous into the broth, cover, and remove from heat. Let sit for 5 minutes.

8. Stir the cooked couscous into the cooked vegetables and serve hot.

VARIATION: When asparagus isn't in season or for taste preference, zucchini makes a tasty substitute.

Zucchini Croquettes

Yield: 4 servings | Prep Time: 10 minutes | Cooking Time: 6 minutes zucchini, 11–12 minutes croquettes | Total Time: 27–28 minutes

These delicate veggie croquettes have a very light texture and a bold flavor. They work equally well as a side dish or an appetizer anytime.

oil for misting or cooking spray

2 cups shredded zucchini

$1/2$ cup leftover mashed potatoes

2 tablespoons grated Parmesan-style topping

$1/4$ teaspoon garlic powder

$1/4$ teaspoon salt

1–2 tablespoons potato starch

$1/2$ cup panko breadcrumbs

1. Spray the air fryer baking pan with oil or cooking spray.

2. Add the shredded zucchini and cook at 390°F for 3 minutes.

3. Stir the zucchini, mist it with oil, and cook for 3 more minutes to soften.

4. In a large bowl, add the cooked zucchini, mashed potatoes, Parmesan topping, garlic powder, salt, and 1 tablespoon of potato starch. Stir together.

5. In a food processor, process half of the veggie mixture for about 1 minute or just long enough to make the mixture very smooth.

6. Transfer the processed mixture back to the remaining zucchini-potato mixture and stir. If the mixture seems too liquid, stir in the other tablespoon of potato starch.

7. Place the panko crumbs in a shallow dish.

8. Shape the vegetable mixture into 12 balls and carefully roll each in panko crumbs.

9. Mist the croquettes with oil, place them in the air fryer basket, and cook at 390°F for 11 to 12 minutes, or until they're golden brown and crispy on the outside.

TIP: To make the coating process easier, drop the veggie mixture by the spoonful directly into the dish with the panko crumbs. Instead of touching the soft croquette with your fingers, push the crumbs around and over it. (Use your fingers like little push brooms.)

SALADS

Broccoli-Tofu Salad

Yield: 4 servings | Prep Time: 50 minutes | Cooking Time: 17–20 minutes | Total Time: 1 hour 7–10 minutes

GLUTEN FREE   TASTER FAVORITE

Air fryers do a great job on tofu, breaded or not, as in this recipe. You do need to make sure it's well drained, though. A tofu press is a great tool to have in your kitchen, but we've included alternative instructions if you don't have one.

Tofu

4 ounces extra-firm tofu

1 teaspoon smoked paprika

1 teaspoon onion powder

$\frac{1}{4}$ teaspoon salt

2 tablespoons cornstarch

1 tablespoon extra-virgin olive oil

Salad

4 cups fresh broccoli, bite-sized pieces

$\frac{1}{2}$ chopped cup red onion, chopped

$\frac{1}{3}$ cup raisins or dried cherries

$\frac{3}{4}$ cup sliced almonds

$\frac{1}{2}$ cup Asian-style salad dressing

1. First drain the tofu. If you have a tofu press, place the tofu in it, press for 30 minutes, and skip to step 3. If not, follow step 2.

2. On a plate, place several folded paper towels. Place the tofu on top, cover with more folded paper towels, and top with a plate. Add canned goods or other heavy items to weight it down. Press the tofu for 30 minutes.

3. While the tofu is draining, in a large bowl, toss together all the salad ingredients. Cover and chill.

4. Cut the drained tofu block into small cubes, about $\frac{1}{4}$-inch thick.

5. In a small bowl, mix together the smoked paprika, onion powder, and salt.

6. Sprinkle the tops and bottoms of the tofu cubes with the smoked paprika mixture.

7. In a small plastic bag or container with lid, add the cornstarch and tofu and shake to coat.

8. In another small plastic bag or container with lid, add the olive oil and coated tofu cubes and shake to coat thoroughly.

9. Cook at 330°F for 17 to 20 minutes, or until the cubes become as crispy as you like.

10. To serve, stir the salad to redistribute dressing, divide among serving plates, and top with the cooked tofu.

NOTE: We recommend Newman's Own Sesame Ginger Dressing for this recipe.

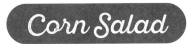

Corn Salad

Yield: 6 servings | Prep Time: 18 minutes | Cooking Time: 10–12 minutes | Total Time: 28–30 minutes

GLUTEN FREE

If you're cooking beans, cook lots and freeze the extras for future meals. This recipe makes good use of those extra or even just leftover beans. Serve this versatile salad as a light lunch, a side dish, or as a dip with Tortilla Strips (page 47).

1 tablespoon light olive oil

½ teaspoon garlic powder

½ teaspoon cumin

2 small ears corn

1 cup cooked black beans

½ cup slivered poblano peppers

½ medium red or white onion

1 small avocado

3 tablespoons lime juice

¼ teaspoon salt

1. In a small bowl, mix the olive oil, garlic powder, and cumin.

2. Remove the husks and silk from the ears of corn.

3. Brush the oil mixture over all surfaces of the corn.

4. Place the corn in the air fryer basket and cook at 390°F for 10 to 12 minutes.

5. While the corn is cooking, slice the poblano peppers into small slivers, ⅛-inch wide, and then dice the onion.

6. When the corn has finished cooking, place the ears on a cutting board, stem end down, and cut or scrape the kernels from the cobs.

7. Dice the avocado into ¼-inch cubes.

8. Toss the corn, beans, peppers, onion, and avocado together with the lime juice and salt.

See insert B7 for recipe photo.

> **TIP:** You can serve this dish warm or chilled, depending on the season or your preference.

Crabless Salad with Pineapple Salsa

Yield: 4 servings | Prep Time: 10 minutes | Cooking Time: 10 minutes | Total Time: 20 minutes

SUPER EASY

After a heavy lunch, you might want to have a light and tasty supper. Crabless Salad suits us perfectly.

2 (8-ounce) packages crabless cakes (10 count)

oil for misting or cooking spray

1 cup minced pineapple

⅓ cup minced red onion

⅓ cup minced bell pepper, any color

4 cups shredded cabbage

1. Mist all sides of the crab cakes with oil or cooking spray and place them in the air fryer basket.

2. Cook at 390°F for 10 minutes, until they turn brown and crisp.

3. Meanwhile, prepare the pineapple, red onion, and bell pepper and stir them together to make the salsa.

4. On each of 4 salad plates, place 1 cup of shredded cabbage.

5. Divide the salsa evenly over the cabbage.

6. Arrange 5 of the cooked cakes on each plate to serve.

NOTE: We recommended Gardein Crabless Cakes for this recipe.

Portabella Salad

Yield: 2 servings | Prep Time: 15 minutes | Cooking Time: 10 minutes | Total Time: 25 minutes

You can double this recipe easily. Cook all the mushrooms at once as long as they don't touch the upper heating element. Total cooking time will take a bit longer, and you'll need to pause several times to rearrange the mushrooms—but otherwise it's a breeze.

Mushrooms

6 ounces portabella mushroom caps (3 caps, about 4½-inches diameter each)

1 tablespoon vegan Worcestershire sauce

¼ teaspoon dry mustard

¼ teaspoon lemon juice

black pepper

1 tablespoon extra-light olive oil

Salad Dressing

6 tablespoons vegan mayonnaise

1 tablespoon almond milk

2 teaspoons prepared horseradish

½ teaspoon coarse brown mustard

½ teaspoon vegan Worcestershire sauce

Salad

4 cups romaine lettuce

6 grape or cherry tomatoes, halved

¼ small red onion, slivered

1. Remove and discard mushroom stems.

2. Clean the mushroom caps and remove the gills.

3. In a small bowl, make a marinade by combining the vegan Worcestershire sauce, mustard, lemon juice, pepper, and oil. Mix well.

4. Brush the marinade onto the mushroom tops. Turn the mushrooms over and brush the stem sides liberally with marinade as well.

5. Place the caps in the air fryer basket, stem side up. Stack them slightly or lean them against the sides of the basket if necessary but leave some space between.

6. Cook at 360°F for 5 minutes.

7. Turn the mushrooms over and cook for 5 more minutes or until done.

8. While the mushrooms cook, make the salad dressing. In a small bowl, combine all dressing ingredients, whisk to mix well, and refrigerate until ready to serve.

9. Cut the mushrooms into bite-size pieces.

10. Divide the greens, tomatoes, and onion slivers between 2 plates. Top with the mushroom pieces and pass the salad dressing at the table.

Potato Salad with Asparagus

Yield: 6–8 servings | Prep Time: 15 minutes | Cooking Time: 12 minutes | Total Time: 27 minutes

GLUTEN FREE **TASTER FAVORITE**

This potato salad is full of flavor. Serve it as a side or make it the main event.

3 medium Yukon Gold potatoes

1 tablespoon light olive oil

1/2 teaspoon thyme

1 1/2 cups asparagus

1/2 medium red onion

salt and pepper

Balsamic Dressing

1 tablespoon light olive oil

2 tablespoons balsamic vinegar

1 tablespoon Dijon mustard

1. Using a vegetable brush, scrub the potatoes under cool running water.

2. Dice the potatoes into 3/4-inch cubes.

3. In a medium bowl, mix the oil and thyme together and toss the potatoes in it.

4. Spoon the potatoes into the air fryer basket, reserving the oil and mixing bowl for later use.

5. Cook potatoes at 390°F for 6 minutes.

6. While the potatoes are cooking, cut the asparagus into 3-inch pieces and then slice the onions thin.

7. Toss the asparagus and onions in the oil remaining in the mixing bowl.

8. Add the coated asparagus and onions and to the potatoes in the air fryer.

9. Cook for 6 more minutes.

10. While the veggies are cooking, make the balsamic dressing by combining all the dressing ingredients in a small bowl.

11. Toss the warm vegetables with the balsamic dressing and cool to lukewarm, stirring occasionally.

12. Season with salt and pepper to taste.

> **TIP:** Don't waste those tough asparagus stems. Save them with other vegetable scraps to make vegetable stock.

Tofu Napa Salad

Yield: 4 servings | Prep Time: 10 minutes, plus 30 minutes marinating | Cooking Time: 10 minutes | Total Time: 50 minutes

GLUTEN FREE

You may think Napa cabbage is only for spring rolls, but it also makes a delicious choice for salad greens. Mildly flavored tofu and tangy mustard dressing set it off nicely.

---

14 ounces firm tofu, pressed

3 tablespoons cornstarch

oil for misting or cooking spray

Marinade

1/2 teaspoon smoked paprika

1/4 teaspoon salt

1/4 teaspoon garlic powder

1/2 teaspoon onion powder

1/8 teaspoon ginger

1 tablespoon extra-light olive oil

Dressing

1 tablespoon coconut sugar

2 tablespoons red wine vinegar

2 tablespoons coarse brown mustard

3 tablespoons extra-light olive oil

Salad

1/4 sweet red bell pepper

1 large Granny Smith apple

8 cups shredded Napa cabbage

> **TIP:** For more crunch, cook as directed above, then continue cooking at 390°F for 5 more minutes or until the tofu is as crispy as you like.

1. Cut the tofu into 1/2-inch cubes.

2. In a plastic bag or a small container with a lid, add the tofu.

3. In a small bowl, combine the marinade ingredients, mix well, and pour over the tofu cubes. Refrigerate for at least 30 minutes or up to overnight.

4. When ready to cook, preheat the air fryer to 390°F.

5. In another plastic bag or container with a lid, add the cornstarch and the marinated tofu cubes and shake to coat lightly.

6. Place the tofu cubes in the air fryer basket, mist them with oil, and cook for 5 minutes.

7. Shake the basket to redistribute the cubes, mist with oil again, and cook for 5 more minutes.

8. Transfer the cubes to a plate to cool slightly.

9. While the tofu is cooking, make the dressing. In a jar or cruet, stir the sugar into the vinegar to dissolve. Add the remaining dressing ingredients and shake vigorously to mix well.

10. Cut the red bell pepper into slivers and core, quarter, and cut the apple crosswise into slices.

11. In a large bowl, toss together the cabbage, bell pepper slivers, apple slices, and dressing.

12. Divide the salad mixture among 4 plates and top with the tofu.

Warm Fruit Salad

Yield: 4–6 servings | Prep Time: 10 minutes | Cooking Time: 9–10 minutes | Total Time: 19–20 minutes

GLUTEN FREE   KID FRIENDLY   SUPER EASY

This versatile dish works well as a side for a wide range of main courses, but it's equally delicious for breakfast or as a not-too-sweet dessert. The air fryer will toast the topping in only a minute, so you don't have to waste time and energy heating up your whole oven.

1/3 cup coconut chips

1/3 cup chopped walnuts

oil for misting or cooking spray

1 cup frozen pineapple, thawed

1 cup frozen peaches, thawed

1 (15-ounce) can dark, sweet pitted cherries, drained

1/4 teaspoon brandy extract

1 small banana

2 tablespoons dried cranberries or raisins

1. Preheat the air fryer to 390°F.

2. Combine the coconut chips and walnuts in the air fryer baking pan, mist with oil, and stir.

3. Cook 1 to 2 minutes to brown. *Watch carefully!* Coconut can go from golden brown to burned black in 30 seconds or less. Pause your air fryer and check frequently to avoid overcooking.

4. Remove the topping from the baking pan and set aside.

5. In the same baking pan, stir together the pineapple, peaches, cherries, and brandy flavoring.

6. Cook the fruit mixture for 4 minutes.

7. Stir and cook for 2 more minutes.

8. Cut the banana into slices and add them to the fruit mixture.

9. Cook for 2 more minutes or until the banana warms.

10. Stir the cranberries or raisins into the warm fruit when ready to serve.

11. Divide the fruit salad among small salad or dessert bowls and sprinkle with the toasted coconut and nuts.

BREADS

Artisan Loaf with Roasted Peppers & Olives

Yield: 8 servings | Prep Time: 25 minutes | Cooking Time: 20–25 minutes | Total Time: 45–50 minutes

White whole wheat flour offers a nice compromise between white flour and heavier whole-grain red wheat. We like a variety of olives in this bread so no one particular taste dominates, but feel free to use your olive or olives of choice. It's easier to buy the roasted red peppers in a jar, packed in water (not oil).

1½ teaspoons coconut sugar

1 cup lukewarm water

1 (¼-ounce) package rapid-rise yeast

1⅓ cups whole-grain white wheat flour

⅛ teaspoon salt

1 teaspoon dried basil

2 teaspoons extra-virgin olive oil

⅓ cup chopped roasted red peppers (from a jar)

⅓ cup minced olives

oil for misting or cooking spray

1. In a medium bowl, mix together the coconut sugar and lukewarm water.

2. Stir in the yeast.

3. Add the flour, salt, basil, and olive oil and beat with a wooden spoon for 2 minutes.

4. Add the peppers and olives. Rather than a stiff dough, you will have a thick batter at this point.

5. Spray or mist the air fryer baking pan with oil, pour in the batter, and smooth the top.

6. Let the batter rise for 15 minutes.

7. Preheat the air fryer to 360°F.

8. Cook the bread for 20 to 25 minutes, until a toothpick inserted in the center of the bread comes out with moist crumbs clinging to it.

9. Let the bread rest in the pan for 10 minutes before turning it out.

> **TIP:** We recommend using King Arthur brand flour for this recipe.

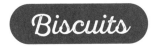

Biscuits

Yield: 4 servings | Prep Time: 10 minutes | Cooking Time: 8–9 minutes | Total Time: 18–19 minutes

GREAT SNACK   KID FRIENDLY   TASTER FAVORITE

Use plain white vinegar in this recipe. It won't affect the taste, but it will curdle the almond milk a bit, which helps create a fluffy texture similar to that of old-fashioned buttermilk biscuits.

6 tablespoons almond milk

1 teaspoon distilled white vinegar

1½ cups all-purpose white flour

2¼ teaspoons baking powder

¼ teaspoon baking soda

¼ teaspoon salt

3 tablespoons cold vegan butter

oil for misting or cooking spray

1 teaspoon melted vegan butter

1. In a small bowl or cup, stir together the almond milk and vinegar.

2. Preheat the air fryer to 390°F.

3. In a medium bowl, combine the flour, baking powder, soda, and salt and stir together.

4. Add the cold vegan butter and, using a pastry blender, cut it into the flour.

5. Pour in the almond milk mixture and stir into a stiff dough.

6. Shape the dough into 4 biscuits about ½-inch thick. If the dough feels too sticky to handle, stir in another tablespoon of flour before shaping.

7. Spray the air fryer basket with oil or nonstick cooking spray.

8. Place all 4 biscuits in the basket, brush the tops with melted butter, and cook for 8 to 9 minutes.

See insert B8 for recipe photo.

Blueberry Muffins

Yield: 8 muffins | Prep Time: 15 minutes | Cooking Time: 9–10 minutes per batch (2 batches) | Total Time: 33–35 minutes

KID FRIENDLY

In this all-time favorite, you get both comfort food and super food. While your taste buds enjoy the flavors, your body will appreciate all the nutrients from the berries.

1½ teaspoons distilled white vinegar

scant ½ cup almond milk

1 tablespoon flaxseed meal

2 tablespoons water

1 cup all-purpose white flour

¼ cup coconut sugar

1 teaspoon baking powder

½ teaspoon baking soda

⅛ teaspoon salt

2 tablespoons coconut oil

½ teaspoon pure vanilla extract

½ cup fresh blueberries

8 foil muffin cups

cooking spray

1. In a measuring cup, add the vinegar.

2. Add enough almond milk to fill to ½ cup.

3. In a small bowl, mix the flaxseed meal and water.

4. Preheat the air fryer to 330°F.

5. In a large bowl, stir together the flour, sugar, baking powder, soda, and salt.

6. Warm the coconut oil just enough to liquefy it. Pour it into the bowl with the flaxseed meal.

7. Add the almond milk and vanilla and stir together.

8. Pour the liquids over the dry ingredients and stir just until moistened. Do not beat.

9. Gently fold in the blueberries.

10. Remove the liners from 8 foil muffin cups and spray the cups with cooking spray.

11. Divide the batter among 8 muffin cups and place 4 muffin cups in the air fryer basket.

12. Cook at 330°F for 9 to 10 minutes.

13. Repeat with the 4 remaining muffins.

Bran Muffins

Yield: 8 muffins | Prep Time: 10 minutes | Cooking Time: 10–11 minutes per batch (2 batches) | Total Time: 30–32 minutes

Molasses and chopped dates add a mild sweetness to these dark bran muffins. They make a filling breakfast food or snack and provide a good source of both fiber and protein.

1 tablespoon Bob's Red Mill egg replacer

2 tablespoons water

$\frac{2}{3}$ cup oat bran

$\frac{1}{2}$ cup all-purpose white flour

1 teaspoon baking powder

$\frac{1}{2}$ teaspoon baking soda

$\frac{1}{8}$ teaspoon salt

$\frac{1}{4}$ cup almond milk

2 tablespoons coconut oil

3 tablespoons molasses

$\frac{1}{2}$ cup chopped dates

8 foil muffin cups

1. Preheat the air fryer to 330°F.

2. In a small cup, mix the egg replacer and water together. Set aside for 1 minute to thicken.

3. In a large bowl, combine the oat bran, flour, baking powder, baking soda, and salt.

4. In another small bowl or saucepan, add the almond milk and coconut oil and warm it just enough barely to melt the oil.

5. Stir in the egg mixture and molasses and blend well.

6. Pour the liquid mixture into the dry ingredients and stir just until moistened. Do not beat.

7. Gently fold in the dates.

8. Place 4 foil muffin cups (no paper liners) in the air fryer basket and fill each one $\frac{3}{4}$ full with batter.

9. Cook for 10 to 11 minutes, until the top springs back when lightly touched and a toothpick inserted in the center comes out clean.

10. Repeat to cook the 4 remaining muffins.

See insert C1 for recipe photo.

> **TIP:** These muffins taste best served warm, and you can reheat leftovers easily in your air fryer in just 1 or 2 minutes at 330°F.

Carrot-Nut Muffins

Yield: 8 muffins | Prep Time: 10 minutes | Cooking Time: 10–12 minutes per batch (2 batches) | Total Time: 30–34 minutes

These super-moist muffins are brimming with healthy ingredients, but your taste buds will think you're indulging in a decadent treat.

¾ cup whole wheat flour

¼ cup oat bran

2 tablespoons flaxseed meal

¼ cup coconut sugar

1 teaspoon baking powder

¼ teaspoon salt

½ teaspoon pumpkin pie spice

¾ cup almond milk

2 tablespoons Date Paste (page 152)

½ teaspoon pure vanilla extract

¾ cup grated carrots

½ cup chopped walnuts

1 tablespoon pumpkin seeds

16 foil muffin cups

cooking spray

1. Preheat the air fryer to 330°F.

2. In a large bowl, stir together the flour, bran, flaxseed meal, sugar, baking powder, salt, and pumpkin pie spice.

3. In a medium bowl, whisk together the milk, Date Paste, and vanilla.

4. Pour the milk mixture into the flour mixture and stir just until the dry ingredients are moistened. Do not beat.

5. Gently stir in the carrots, nuts, and seeds.

6. Remove the paper liners from 16 muffin cups and save for another use. Double up the cups so that you have 8 total and spray them with cooking spray.

7. Place 4 foil cups in the air fryer basket and fill them almost full with batter.

8. Cook at 330°F for 10 to 12 minutes or until a toothpick inserted in the center comes out clean.

9. Repeat steps 7 and 8 to cook the 4 remaining muffins.

Chocolate-Cherry Scones

Yield: 9 scones | Prep Time: 20 minutes | Cooking Time: 8–11 minutes | Total Time: 28–31 minutes

KID FRIENDLY

Who doesn't love chocolate and cherries together? This recipe makes a semi-decadent dessert or a deliciously sweet breakfast—your choice!

oil for misting or cooking spray

2¼ cups self-rising flour, divided

⅓ cup sugar

⅓ cup dried cherries

2 ounces 70 percent cocoa dark chocolate

⅓ cup sliced almonds (optional)

¼ cup vegan butter or coconut oil

1 cup almond milk

1. Spray the air fryer basket with oil or cooking spray.
2. Preheat the air fryer to 360°F.
3. In a medium bowl, stir together 2 cups of flour and the sugar.
4. Using kitchen shears, snip the cherries and chocolate directly into the flour and stir to blend.
5. Stir in the almonds, if using, with the chocolate and cherries.
6. Using a fork, blend the butter or coconut oil into the flour mixture.
7. Stir in the milk.
8. Put the remaining ¼ cup flour on a sheet of wax paper and turn out the dough onto it.
9. Knead lightly by folding and turning 6 to 8 times.
10. Pat the dough into a 6 x 6-inch square.
11. Cut the dough into 9 equal-size pieces and lay the squares in the basket. Arrange them close together but not quite touching.
12. Cook at 360°F for 8 to 11 minutes, until lightly browned.

Cinnamon Biscuits

Yield: 8 small biscuits | Prep Time: 12 minutes | Cooking Time: 9–11 minutes | Total Time: 21–23 minutes

KID FRIENDLY   TASTER FAVORITE

We prefer these rich cinnamon biscuits plain, but you can add a dab of vegan butter or a drizzle of maple syrup if you like. If you have a serious sweet tooth, try topping them with a maple or sugar glaze.

3 tablespoons coconut sugar

¾ teaspoon cinnamon

1½ cups all-purpose white flour

2¼ teaspoons baking powder

¼ teaspoon baking soda

3 tablespoons cold vegan butter

½ cup cold vegan sour cream

1 teaspoon almond milk or water

additional almond milk

1 tablespoon melted vegan butter

cooking spray

TIP: For this recipe, we used Tofutti brand vegan sour cream, which is extremely stiff when cold, making it very difficult to stir into dry ingredients. If your brand of sour cream is softer, thinning it (step 6) may not be necessary. Don't use room-temperature sour cream for this recipe.

1. Preheat the air fryer to 360°F.

2. In a large bowl, mix the sugar and cinnamon. Reserve 2 teaspoons and set aside for sprinkling at the end.

3. To the remaining cinnamon sugar, add the flour, baking powder, and baking soda and stir.

4. Using a pastry blender, cut the cold butter into the dry ingredients.

5. In a small bowl, mix the cold sour cream with 1 teaspoon of milk or water to thin it. (See note below.)

6. Add the sour cream to the dry ingredients and stir until a stiff dough begins to form. If the dough is very dry, stir in up to 1 more tablespoon of almond milk, 1 teaspoon at a time. The dough should be mixed well but still feel slightly crumbly.

7. Turn out the dough on wax paper and knead it just enough to work the remaining dry crumbs into the dough, about 30 to 60 seconds.

8. Divide the dough into 8 portions and shape those into biscuits, each about 2 inches in diameter.

9. Brush the tops of the biscuits liberally with the melted vegan butter, then sprinkle with the reserved cinnamon sugar.

10. Spray the air fryer basket with nonstick cooking spray.

11. Place all 8 biscuits in the air fryer basket and cook at 360°F for 9 to 11 minutes, until done inside.

Cinnamon Pecan Bread

Yield: 8 servings | Prep Time: 25 minutes | Cooking Time: 20–25 minutes | Total Time: 45–50 minutes

Cinnamon bread is one of our favorites. Feel free to leave out the pecans or use walnuts or your favorite nuts instead.

3 tablespoons coconut sugar

1 cup lukewarm water

1 (¼-ounce) package rapid-rise yeast

1⅓ cups whole-grain white wheat flour

2 teaspoons light olive oil

½ teaspoon salt

2 teaspoons cinnamon

½ cup chopped pecans

oil for misting or cooking spray

1. In a medium bowl, stir together the coconut sugar and water.

2. Stir in the yeast.

3. Add the flour, oil, salt, and cinnamon and stir until well blended.

4. Stir in the pecans. You will have a thick batter rather than a stiff dough.

5. Spray the air fryer baking pan and pour the batter into it.

6. Set aside to rise for 15 minutes.

7. Preheat the air fryer to 360°F.

8. Cook for 20 to 25 minutes, until a toothpick pushed into the center comes out with soft crumbs clinging to it.

Cranberry Muffins

Yield: 8 muffins | Prep Time: 10 minutes | Cooking Time: 9–10 minutes per batch (2 batches) | Total Time: 28–30 minutes

TASTER FAVORITE

The nutty crunch of oat bran in this tasty and nutritious recipe offers a perfect partner for the chewy dried cranberries.

1½ teaspoons distilled white vinegar

scant ½ cup almond milk

1 tablespoon flaxseed meal

2 tablespoons water

⅔ cup oat bran

½ cup all-purpose white flour

¼ cup coconut sugar

1 teaspoon baking powder

½ teaspoon baking soda

⅛ teaspoon salt

2 tablespoons extra-light olive oil

¼ cup dried cranberries

8 foil muffin cups

cooking spray

1. In a measuring cup, add the vinegar.

2. Add enough almond milk to measure ½ cup.

3. In a small bowl, mix the flaxseed meal and water and set aside.

4. Preheat the air fryer to 330°F.

5. In a large bowl, stir together the oat bran, flour, sugar, baking powder, baking soda, and salt.

6. Add the almond milk mixture and olive oil to the flaxseed water and stir together.

7. Pour the liquid ingredients over the dry ingredients and stir just until moistened. Do not beat.

8. Gently fold in the cranberries.

9. Remove the liners from 8 foil muffin cups and spray the cups with cooking spray.

10. Divide the batter among the muffin cups.

11. Place 4 muffin cups in the air fryer basket and cook at 330°F for 9 to 10 minutes.

12. Repeat with the 4 remaining muffins.

See insert C2 for recipe photo.

Cranberry-Orange Scones

Yield: 9 scones | Prep Time: 20 minutes | Cooking Time: 8–11 minutes | Total Time: 28–31 minutes

TASTER FAVORITE

We love the taste combination of cranberries and orange. These will be a big hit on your breakfast table or the next time you have people over for tea.

oil for misting or cooking spray

2¼ cups whole-grain white wheat flour, divided

2 teaspoons baking powder

⅓ cup coconut sugar

¼ cup minced dried cranberries

1 teaspoon grated orange peel

¼ cup coconut oil

¾ cup almond or coconut milk

¼ cup fresh squeezed orange juice

1. Spray the air fryer basket with oil or cooking spray.

2. Preheat the air fryer to 360°F.

3. In a medium bowl, stir together 2 cups of flour, baking powder, coconut sugar, cranberries, and orange peel.

4. Using a fork, blend the coconut oil into the flour mixture.

5. Stir in the milk and orange juice to form a soft dough.

6. Put the remaining ¼ cup of flour on a sheet of wax paper and turn out the dough onto it.

7. Knead lightly by folding and turning 6 to 8 times.

8. Pat the dough into a 6 x 6-inch square.

9. Cut the dough into 9 equal pieces and lay the squares in the basket. Arrange them close together but not quite touching.

10. Cook for 8 to 11 minutes, until lightly browned.

NOTE: We recommend King Arthur brand flour for this recipe.

Creamy Chive Biscuits

Yield: 4 servings (8 small biscuits) | Prep Time: 10 minutes | Cooking Time: 10 minutes | Total Time: 20 minutes

TASTER FAVORITE

These savory biscuits pair well with almost any soup, salad, or main dish. If you love bread (like we love bread), you can make a meal of them!

1 cup self-rising flour

1 teaspoon dried chopped chives

½ teaspoon garlic powder

2 tablespoons cold vegan butter

½ cup cold vegan sour cream

1 teaspoon almond milk or water

cooking spray

oil for misting

1. Preheat the air fryer to 330°F.

2. In a medium bowl, combine the flour, chives, and garlic and stir them together.

3. Using a pastry blender, cut the cold butter into the dry ingredients.

4. In a small bowl, mix the vegan sour cream with 1 teaspoon of milk or water to thin it. (See note below.)

5. Add the sour cream to the dry ingredients and stir until a stiff dough begins to form. If needed, stir in up to 1 more tablespoon of almond milk, 1 teaspoon at a time. The dough should be mixed well but still feel slightly crumbly.

6. Turn out the dough on a sheet of wax paper and knead for 30 to 60 seconds, just long enough to work the remaining dry crumbs into the dough.

7. Divide the dough into 8 portions and shape them into biscuits about 2 inches in diameter.

8. Spray the air fryer basket with nonstick cooking spray.

9. Place all 8 biscuits in the air fryer basket and cook for 8 minutes.

10. Mist the tops of the biscuits with oil and cook for 2 more minutes or until done inside.

TIP: For this recipe, we used Tofutti brand vegan sour cream, which is extremely stiff when cold, making it very difficult to stir into dry ingredients. If your brand of sour cream is softer, thinning it (step 5) may not be necessary. Don't use room-temperature sour cream for this recipe.

Tropical Muffins

Yield: 8 muffins | Prep Time: 15 minutes | Cooking Time: 9–10 minutes per batch (2 batches) | Total Time: 33–35 minutes

TASTER FAVORITE

For this recipe, we used packaged fruit cups for convenience, but you certainly can use fresh instead. You'll need ⅓ cup of small pineapple chunks and ½ cup of freshly squeezed juice.

1 tablespoon flaxseed meal

2 tablespoons water

1 (4-ounce) fruit cup pineapple tidbits, with juice

1 cup 2 tablespoons flour

2 tablespoons coconut sugar

1 teaspoon baking powder

½ teaspoon baking soda

⅛ teaspoon salt

2 tablespoons coconut oil

½ teaspoon pure vanilla extract

¼ cup chopped macadamia nuts

¼ cup coconut chips

8 foil muffin cups

cooking spray

1. In a small bowl, mix the flaxseed meal and water together and set aside.

2. Preheat the air fryer to 330°F.

3. Drain the pineapple, reserving the juice to a measuring cup. Press the pineapple tidbits lightly to remove excess moisture—but don't crush them.

4. In a large bowl, stir together the flour, sugar, baking powder, baking soda, and salt.

5. Warm the coconut oil just enough to liquefy it.

6. Add enough water to the reserved pineapple juice to measure ½ cup, then pour the juice into the flaxseed water.

7. Add the oil and vanilla to the flaxseed juice mixture and stir together.

8. Pour the liquid ingredients over the dry ingredients and stir just until moistened. Do not beat.

9. Add the nuts, coconut chips, and pineapple tidbits to the batter and gently fold them in.

10. Remove the liners from 8 foil muffin cups and spray the cups with cooking spray.

11. Divide the batter among the muffin cups.

12. Place 4 muffin cups in the air fryer basket and cook for 9 to 10 minutes.

13. Repeat with the 4 remaining muffins.

DESSERTS

Amaretto Poached Pears

Yield: 3–4 servings | Prep Time: 10 minutes | Cooking Time: 15 minutes | Total Time: 25 minutes

We like to spoon these pears and their flavorsome liquid over slices of Chocolate Cake (page 141). A dollop of whipped coconut cream transforms them into an extra-special dessert.

½ cup amaretto liqueur

½ cup water

2 fresh pears

1. In the air fryer baking pan, pour the amaretto and water.

2. Cut the pears in half lengthwise.

3. Peel and core the pears, then slice them crosswise into ½-inch slices.

4. Stir the pears into the diluted amaretto.

5. Cook at 360°F for 15 minutes, until the pear slices become tender.

6. Cool to room temperature or chill in syrup.

Apple Pies

Yield: 12 pies | Prep Time: 30 minutes | Cooking Time: 18–20 minutes per batch (3 batches) | Total Time: 1 hour 24–30 minutes

KID FRIENDLY   TASTER FAVORITE

Fried pies are a favorite treat from childhood and for childhood. Serve them warm or at room temperature with or without a side of nondairy frozen dessert.

Dough

2¼ cups self-rising flour, divided

¼ cup all-vegetable shortening

¾ cup almond milk

Filling

4 cups peeled, cored, and diced apples

1 tablespoon lemon juice

1 cup sugar

1 tablespoon cornstarch

1 teaspoon cinnamon

oil for misting or cooking spray

1. In a medium bowl, add 2 cups of the flour.

2. Using a pastry blender, cut the shortening into the flour.

3. Stir in the almond milk and set the dough aside while you prepare the apples.

4. Dice the apples into ¼-inch cubes, place them in another medium bowl, add the lemon juice to prevent browning, and stir to coat evenly.

5. In a small bowl, mix the sugar, cornstarch, and cinnamon.

6. Pour the dry ingredients over the apples and stir to coat.

7. Sprinkle remaining ¼ cup flour on a sheet of wax paper.

8. Divide the dough into 12 equal-size balls.

9. On flour-covered wax paper, roll each ball into a thin circle about 5 inches in diameter.

10. Spoon approximately 1½ tablespoons of apple filling onto one side of a dough circle.

11. With a finger dipped in water, moisten the inside edge of the dough circle all around.

12. Fold the dough over to make a half-moon, seal, and crimp the edges with a fork.

13. Repeat steps 10 through 12 with 3 more dough circles.

14. Mist each pie on both sides with oil or cooking spray and place the pies in the air fryer basket.

15. Cook 4 pies at a time at 360°F for 18 to 20 minutes, until they turn light golden brown.

16. While each batch is cooking, repeat steps 10 through 12 (twice) to make the remaining pies.

See insert C3 for recipe photo.

Apple Wedgies

Yield: 4 servings | Prep Time: 10 minutes | Cooking Time: 5 minutes | Total Time: 15 minutes

FAST   GREAT SNACK   KID FRIENDLY

Serve these for a hearty snack or a light dessert. They taste best when hot, but it's fine to cook them early because air fryers do a beautiful job of reheating fried foods.

---

1 tablespoon Bob's Red Mill egg replacer

5 tablespoons water

¼ cup panko breadcrumbs

¼ cup finely chopped peanuts

1 teaspoon coconut sugar

1 teaspoon cocoa powder

1 teaspoon cinnamon

¼ cup potato starch

1 medium Granny Smith apple

oil for misting or cooking spray

1. In a shallow dish, mix the egg replacer and water and set aside to thicken.

2. In another shallow dish, mix together the breadcrumbs, peanuts, sugar, cocoa, and cinnamon.

3. In a resealable plastic bag or a container with a lid, place the potato starch.

4. Preheat the air fryer to 390°F.

5. Cut the apple into small wedges. The thickest edge should be no more than 3/8- to 1/2-inch thick. Cut away the core but don't peel.

6. Place the apple wedges in the potato starch and shake to coat.

7. Dip the wedges in egg wash, shake off the excess, and roll them in the crumb mixture.

8. Spray the wedges with oil or cooking spray, place them in the air fryer basket in a single layer, and cook for 5 minutes or until they turn brown and crispy. The cocoa will make the coating look dark, but you'll see the peanut chunks turn golden brown.

9. Serve hot.

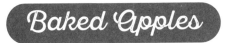

Baked Apples

Yield: 6 apple halves | Prep Time: 10 minutes | Cooking Time: 20 minutes | Total Time: 30 minutes

GLUTEN FREE   KID FRIENDLY

Enjoy this traditional autumn comfort food for a nice light dessert or as a breakfast treat alongside the fried Oatmeal Bars (page 8).

---

3 small honey crisp or other baking apples

3 tablespoons chopped pecans

3 tablespoons pure maple syrup

1 tablespoon vegan butter, divided

1. Pour ½ cup of water into the drawer of the air fryer.

2. Wash and dry the apples and cut each in half.

3. Core the halves and remove about a tablespoon of the apple flesh to make a cavity to hold the pecans.

4. Place the apple halves in the air fryer basket, cut side up.

5. Into the cavity of each apple, spoon 1½ teaspoons of pecans and ½ tablespoon maple syrup.

6. Top each apple half with ½ teaspoon vegan butter.

7. Cook at 360°F for 20 minutes or until the apples become soft and tender.

Banana Bread Pudding

Yield: 1 (6 x 6-inch) loaf (4 to 6 servings) | Prep Time: 10 minutes | Cooking Time: 20–22 minutes | Total Time: 30–32 minutes

For maximum flavor in this recipe, use extremely overripe bananas. The goal is to bake this dish until barely done and still very moist—but really you can't go wrong. If you overcook, it may have a consistency more like a quick bread, but it still will taste wonderful.

1 tablespoon Bob's Red Mill egg replacer

2 tablespoons water

cooking spray

1 cup all-purpose white flour

1 teaspoon baking powder

¼ teaspoon salt

¾ cup mashed ripe banana

¼ cup peanut butter

¼ cup almond milk

¼ cup pure maple syrup

2 tablespoons coconut oil

½ teaspoon pure vanilla extract

1. In a small bowl, mix the egg replacer and water and set aside for 1 minute to thicken.

2. Preheat the air fryer to 330°F.

3. Spray a 6 x 6-inch baking dish lightly with cooking spray.

4. In a medium bowl, mix together the flour, baking powder, and salt.

5. In a separate mixing bowl, combine the banana, peanut butter, milk, maple syrup, coconut oil, vanilla, and egg mixture and mix well.

6. Gently stir the banana mixture into the dry ingredients. Blend well but don't beat. The batter will feel very thick.

7. Spread the batter evenly in the prepared baking dish and cook for 20 to 22 minutes.

8. The pudding is done when the top has browned and feels firm when pressed with the back of a spoon.

Cherry-Berry Crisp

Yield: 4 servings | Prep Time: 10 minutes | Cooking Time: 7–9 minutes | Total Time: 17–19 minutes

GLUTEN FREE   GREAT SNACK   TASTER FAVORITE

This old-fashioned crisp will satisfy your sweet tooth without being too decadent. Its crunchy topping has a great nutty taste and provides some fiber too.

Filling

cooking spray

1 (10-ounce) bag frozen cherries, thawed and undrained

1 cup fresh blueberries

¼ cup coconut sugar

2 tablespoons amaretto liqueur

Topping

2 tablespoons oats

2 tablespoons oat bran

¼ cup cooked quinoa

2 tablespoons sliced almonds

2 tablespoons coconut sugar

2 teaspoons coconut oil

1. Preheat the air fryer to 360°F.

2. Spray the air fryer baking pan with nonstick cooking spray.

3. Combine all filling ingredients in the baking pan and stir well.

4. In a medium bowl, combine all of the topping ingredients and mix until the oil is distributed evenly and the mixture is crumbly.

5. Spoon the topping evenly over the filling in the pan.

6. Cook for 7 to 9 minutes or until the crumb topping turns golden brown and crispy.

Chocolate Cake

Yield: 8 servings | Prep Time: 10 minutes | Cooking Time: 25–30 minutes | Total Time: 35–40 minutes

GREAT SNACK   KID FRIENDLY

This quick-to-make cake is easy as—well, pie.

---

oil for misting or cooking spray

1 tablespoon Bob's Red Mill egg replacer

2 tablespoons water

$\frac{1}{2}$ cup sugar

$\frac{1}{4}$ cup self-rising flour, plus 3 tablespoons

3 tablespoons cocoa

$\frac{1}{4}$ teaspoon baking soda

$\frac{1}{4}$ teaspoon salt

2 tablespoons vegan oil

1 (5.3-ounce) container vegan vanilla yogurt

$\frac{1}{4}$ cup nut milk of choice

1. Preheat the air fryer to 330°F.

2. Spray the baking pan with oil or cooking spray and set aside.

3. In a medium bowl, using a wire whisk, whisk together the egg replacer and water.

4. Add the remaining ingredients and whisk until smooth.

5. Pour the batter into the air fryer baking pan and cook for 25 to 30 minutes, until a toothpick inserted into the center comes out clean.

6. Let the cake rest for 10 minutes before removing it from the pan.

See insert C4 for recipe photo.

Coconut Pound Cake with Pineapple-Lime Topping

Yield: 8 servings | Prep Time: 10 minutes | Cooking Time: 30–35 minutes | Total Time: 40–45 minutes

TASTER FAVORITE

We Southerners love our pound cake. This one is delicious on its own, but the Pineapple-Lime Topping kicks it up a notch.

---

cooking spray

1 tablespoon Bob's Red Mill egg replacer

2 tablespoons water

½ cup sugar

1½ cups self-rising flour

2 tablespoons coconut oil

1 cup coconut milk

½ cup unsweetened flaked coconut

Pineapple Lime Topping

1 (8-ounce) can crushed pineapple in juice, drained

1 teaspoon grated lime zest

1 tablespoon lime juice

1¼ cups sugar

1. Preheat the air fryer to 330°F.

2. Spray the air fryer baking pan with nonstick spray and set aside.

3. In a medium bowl, using a wire whisk, whisk together the egg replacer and water.

4. Add the sugar, flour, coconut oil, and coconut milk and whisk until blended.

5. Stir in the coconut.

6. Pour the batter into the prepared pan and cook for 30 to 35 minutes, until a toothpick inserted into the center comes out with soft crumbs attached.

7. Let the cake rest in the pan for 10 minutes before removing it.

8. While the cake is baking, prepare the topping. In a small saucepan over medium-high heat, combine all of the topping ingredients.

9. Bring the topping to a boil, stirring constantly, boil for 1 minute and then remove from the heat.

10. Let the topping cool and serve it at room temperature.

See insert C5 for recipe photo of the pound cake.

> **VARIATION:** Instead of the Pineapple-Lime Topping, the pound cake also tastes great with Strawberry Sauce (page 148).

Dundee Cake

Yield: 8 servings | Prep Time: 16 minutes | Cooking Time: 30 minutes | Total Time: 46 minutes

Dundee is a Scottish fruit cake often served at teatime. Our Scottish Aunt Margaret says tea always should be served at 4:00 P.M., but this cake tastes good at any time of day. Try it for breakfast with a proper "cuppa."

cooking spray

2 tablespoons Bob's Red Mill egg replacer

4 tablespoons water

4 tablespoons coconut oil

½ cup sugar

1 cup dried currants

⅓ cup slivered almonds

1 tablespoon grated orange peel

1 tablespoon grated lemon peel

1 cup self-rising flour

½ cup almond flour

2 tablespoons orange juice, orange liqueur, or brandy

1. Spray the air fryer baking pan with nonstick cooking spray.

2. Preheat the air fryer to 330°F.

3. In a large bowl, mix together the egg replacer and water.

4. Stir in the coconut oil and sugar and beat until smooth.

5. Add flours, almonds, currants, lemon and orange peels, and orange juice or liqueur or brandy.

6. Pour the batter into the air fryer baking pan, smoothing the top.

7. Cook for 30 minutes, until a toothpick inserted into the center comes out with moist crumbs.

Gingerbread

Yield: 1 (6-inch x 6-inch) loaf (4 to 8 servings) | Prep Time: 5 minutes | Cooking Time: 20 minutes | Total Time: 25 minutes

GREAT SNACK   TASTER FAVORITE

Warm or cold, gingerbread makes a nice dessert when served perfectly plain. You also can top it with sliced fruit or cut it into cubes for layering in a pretty parfait with vegan vanilla ice cream.

1½ teaspoons lemon juice

scant ½ cup almond milk

1 tablespoon Bob's Red Mill egg replacer

2 tablespoons water

cooking spray

1 cup all-purpose white flour

2 tablespoons coconut sugar

¾ teaspoon ground ginger

¼ teaspoon cinnamon

1 teaspoon baking powder

½ teaspoon baking soda

⅛ teaspoon salt

¼ cup molasses

2 tablespoons extra-light olive oil

1 teaspoon pure vanilla extract

1. Pour the lemon juice into a glass measuring cup.

2. Add enough almond milk to measure ½ cup.

3. In a small cup, mix the egg replacer and water and set aside.

4. Preheat the air fryer to 330°F.

5. Spray a 6 x 6-inch baking dish lightly with cooking spray.

6. In a medium bowl, mix together all of the dry ingredients.

7. Add the molasses, olive oil, vanilla extract, and egg replacer mixture to the almond milk and stir until well mixed.

8. Pour the liquid mixture into the dry ingredients and stir until well blended.

9. Pour the batter into the air fryer baking dish and cook for 20 minutes or until a toothpick inserted into the center of the loaf comes out clean.

Peach Fried Pies

Yield: 12 pies | Prep Time: 30 minutes | Cooking Time: 18–20 minutes per batch (3 batches) | Total Time: 84–90 minutes

When peaches ripen in the summer, we start to crave anything made with them. These air-fried pies will do an excellent job of satisfying your summer sweet tooth.

Dough

2 cups self-rising flour

¼ cup all-vegetable shortening

¾ cup almond milk

Filling

¼ cup sugar

1 tablespoon cornstarch

3½ cups diced fresh peaches

½ cup dried cherries

½ cup sliced almonds

1 tablespoon lemon juice

¼–½ cup all-purpose white flour for work surface

oil for misting or cooking spray

1. Pour the flour into a large bowl and, using a pastry blender, cut the shortening into it.

2. Stir in the almond milk until a soft dough forms and set aside.

3. In a separate bowl, stir the filling ingredients together and set aside.

4. Divide the dough into 12 equal-size portions and roll them into balls.

5. On a sheet of wax paper, sprinkle 1 tablespoon of flour.

6. On the wax paper with flour, roll one ball of dough out to a circle about 4½ to 5 inches in diameter. Use additional flour as needed to prevent the dough from sticking.

7. Place a heaping tablespoon of filling on the dough.

8. With a pastry brush or your finger dipped in water, moisten the inside edge of the dough all around.

9. Fold the dough over to make a half-moon shape, press to seal it, and use a fork to crimp the edges shut.

10. Repeat steps 6 through 9 to make 3 more pies.

11. Mist both sides of the pies with oil or cooking spray and place in the air fryer basket.

12. Cook at 360°F for 18 to 20 minutes, until the crust lightly browns.

13. Repeat steps 6–12 twice more to make the remaining pies.

Peach Pudding Cake

Yield: 8 servings | Prep Time: 10 minutes | Cooking Time: 35 minutes | Total Time: 45 minutes

We love the moist richness of this cake. It doesn't need anything else to make it taste better, but fresh raspberries and whipped coconut cream make this a truly heavenly treat.

---

1 (8-ounce) can diced peaches packed in juice, drained

oil for misting or cooking spray

1 tablespoon Bob's Red Mill egg replacer

2 tablespoons water

1 cup self-rising flour

¼ teaspoon baking soda

½ cup sugar

2 tablespoons oil

1 (5.3-ounce) container vegan peach yogurt

¼ cup almond milk

¼ teaspoon almond extract

1. Preheat the air fryer to 330°F.

2. On several layers of paper towels, place the drained peaches in a single layer and top with more paper towels to remove the excess moisture.

3. Spray the air fryer baking pan with oil or cooking spray.

4. In a medium bowl, using a wire whisk, mix the egg replacer with the water.

5. Add the remaining ingredients, including the peaches, and whisk until well mixed.

6. Pour the batter into the air fryer baking pan and cook for 35 minutes or until a toothpick inserted into the center of the cake comes out clean.

7. Let the cake rest for 10 minutes before removing it from the baking pan.

Peaches Poached in Raspberry Syrup

Yield: 6 servings | Prep Time: 20 minutes | Cooking Time: 15 minutes | Total Time: 35 minutes

GLUTEN FREE **TASTER FAVORITE**

You can enjoy these peaches warm, but chilled poached peaches taste divine when spooned over nondairy frozen dessert with a few fresh raspberries for garnish.

---

1 (6-ounce) package frozen raspberries, thawed

½ cup sugar

5 cups water, divided (room temperature)

2 pounds fresh peaches

1 tablespoon lemon juice

1. In a small saucepan over medium-high heat, stir together the raspberries, sugar, and ½ cup water.

2. Bring the raspberries to a boil and cook until the sugar dissolves.

3. While the raspberry syrup is cooking, prepare the peaches. In a large bowl, pour 4 cups of water and the lemon juice.

4. Cut a deep slice off one side of a peach, cutting close to the pit from stem end to blossom end.

5. Turn and make the same cut on the other side of the peach. Cut those two slices in half lengthwise.

6. Cut slices from the two remaining sides of the peach.

7. Peel the peach slices and drop them in the bowl of water.

8. Repeat steps 4 through 7 with the remaining peaches.

9. Drain the peaches and spoon them into the air fryer baking pan.

10. Pour the boiling raspberry syrup over the peaches.

11. Cook at 360°F for 10 minutes.

12. Stir and cook for an additional 5 minutes.

13. Cool to lukewarm and chill if desired.

> **TIP:** You will have *way* more syrup for these than you can eat with the peaches. Not to worry: The syrup tastes utterly delicious when stirred into iced tea or lemonade or blended into smoothies.

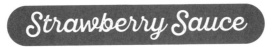

Strawberry Sauce

Yield: 6–8 servings | Prep Time: 10 minutes | Cooking Time: 15 minutes | Total Time: 25 minutes

GLUTEN FREE   KID FRIENDLY   SUPER EASY

Spoon this delectable sauce over slices of Coconut Pound Cake (page 142) for a very special dessert.

1 pound fresh strawberries, coarsely chopped

½ teaspoon grated orange rind

1 teaspoon orange liqueur

½ cup sugar

1. In the air fryer baking pan, stir together the strawberries, orange rind, orange liqueur, and sugar.

2. Cook at 390°F for 5 minutes.

3. Stir and cook for 10 more minutes.

See insert C5 for recipe photo.

NOTE: We recommended Grand Marnier or Cointreau for this recipe.

TIP: If your strawberries are very tart, add up to an additional ½ cup of sugar.

THIS & THAT

Cajun Seasoning Mix

Yield: ¾ cup | Prep Time: 5 minutes | Total Time: 5 minutes

FAST   GLUTEN FREE   SUPER EASY

A sprinkle of our Cajun seasoning on just about anything will make you long for a visit to southern Louisiana.

3 tablespoons paprika

2 tablespoons cayenne pepper

2 tablespoons dried oregano

2 tablespoons garlic powder

2 tablespoons onion powder

2 tablespoons thyme

In a small bowl, stir together all ingredients. Store in an airtight container.

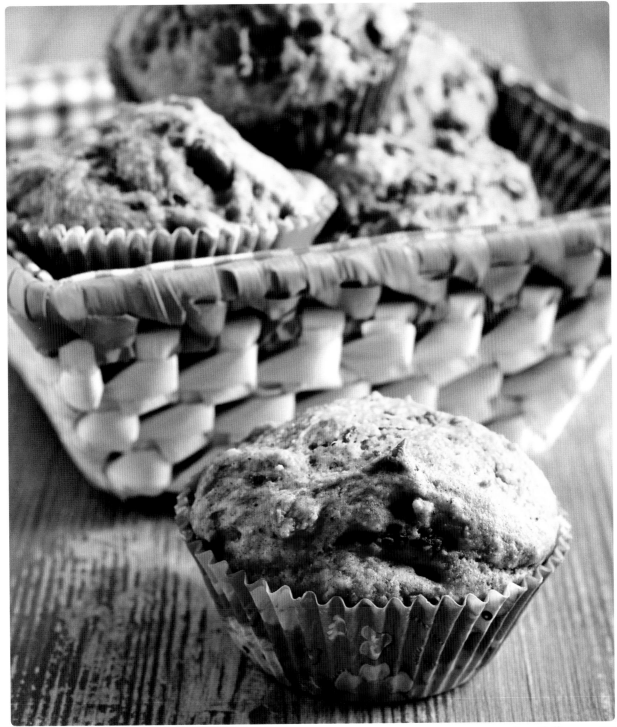

Bran Muffins, page 125

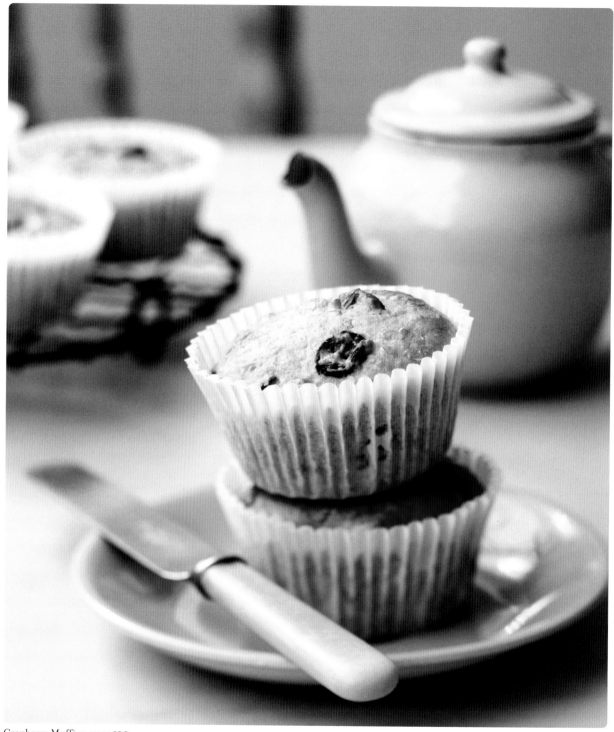

Cranberry Muffins, page 130

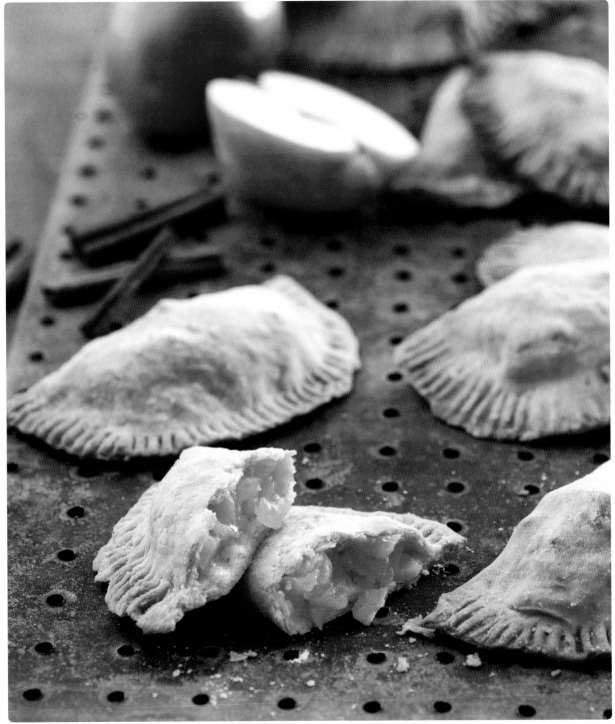

Apple Pies, page 136

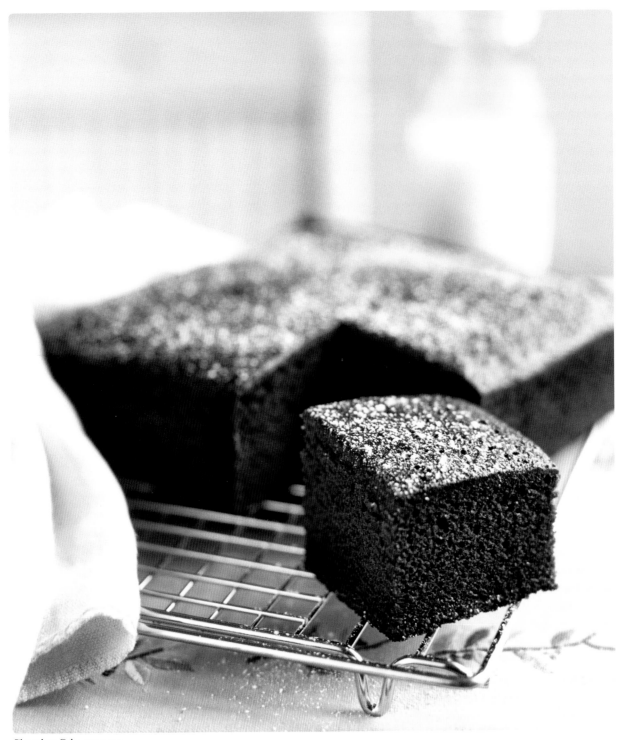

Chocolate Cake, page 141

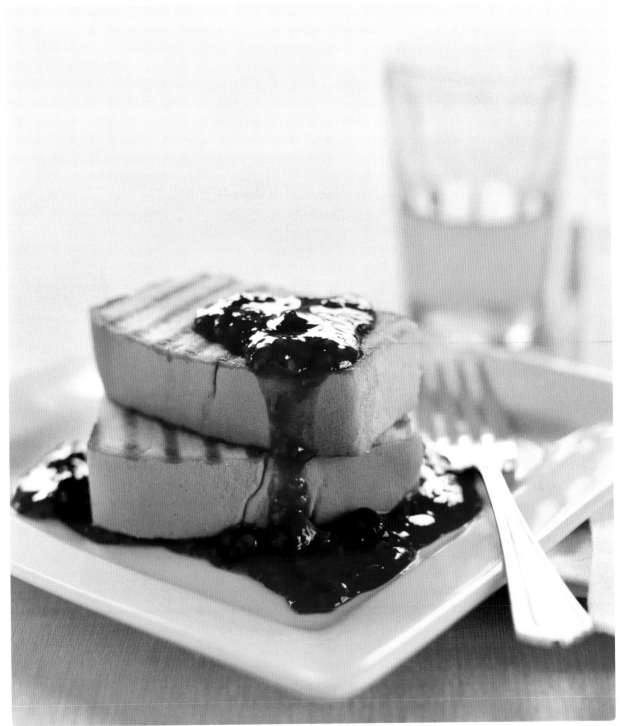

Coconut Pound Cake with Strawberry Sauce, pages 142 and 148

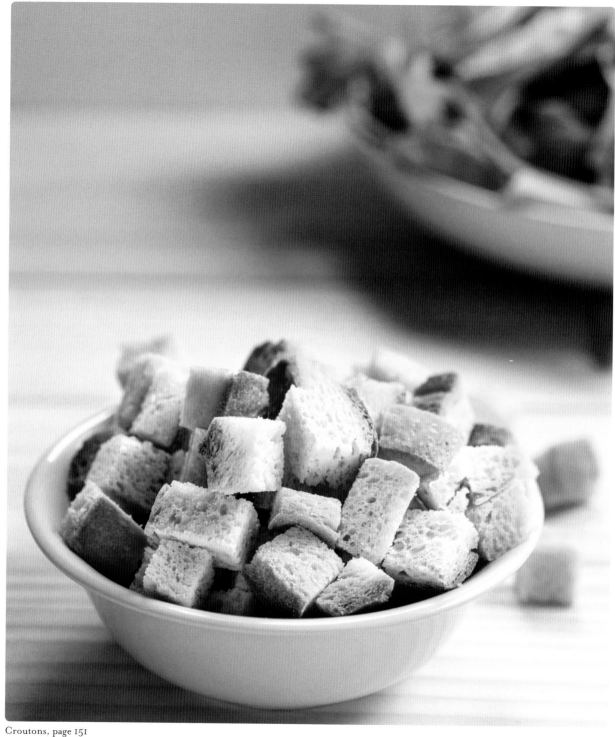

Croutons, page 151

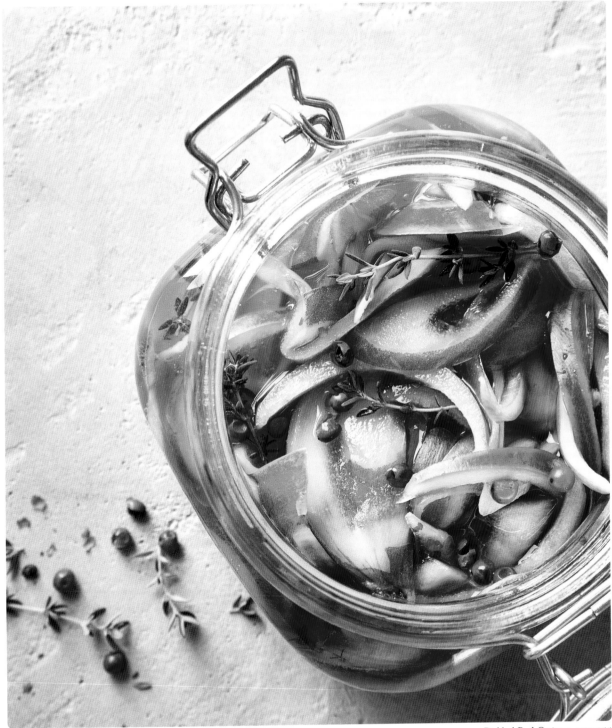

Pickled Red Onions, page 155

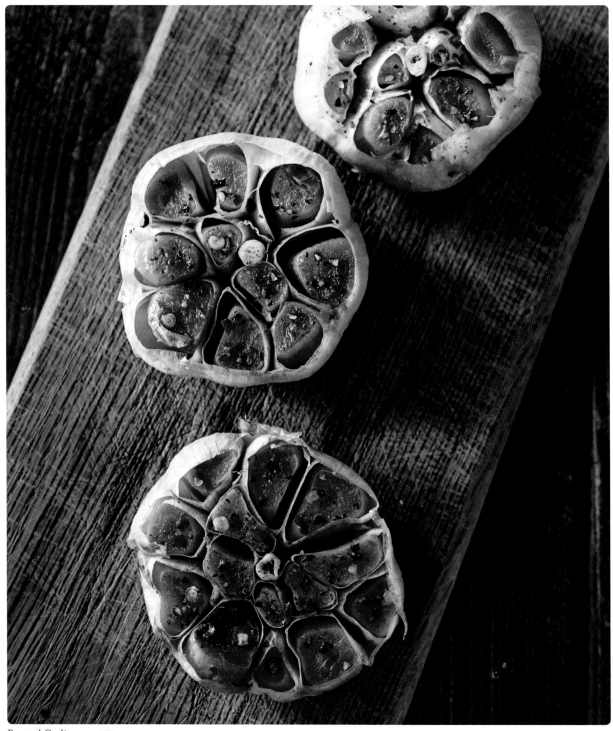

Roasted Garlic, page 157

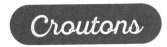

Croutons

Yield: 2 cups | Prep Time: 10 minutes | Cooking Time: 6 minutes | Total Time: 16 minutes

SUPER EASY

Homemade croutons are so easy to make and a great way to use stale bread. They're also healthier than many packaged varieties because you have complete control over the ingredients.

---

1 tablespoon vegan butter

1 tablespoon extra-light olive oil

½ teaspoon garlic powder or other seasoning (optional)

1 small loaf bread, about 8 ounces

1. In a small saucepan over low heat, cook the butter until it begins to brown.

2. Stir in the oil and seasoning, if using. Set aside while you prepare the bread.

3. Cut the bread into ¾-inch cubes.

4. In a large bowl, place the cubed bread, drizzle the oil mixture over the cubes, and stir until well coated.

5. Place the cubes in the air fryer basket and cook at 390°F for 3 minutes.

6. Stir and cook for 3 more minutes or until the croutons turn golden brown and crunchy.

See insert C6 for recipe photo.

VARIATIONS: For light and airy croutons, use French bread. For denser croutons, try ciabatta. Artisan breads also work very well and make for tasty croutons without any extra seasoning.

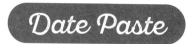

Date Paste

Yield: 1½ cups | Prep Time: 8 hours 5 minutes | Total Time: 8 hours 5 minutes

GLUTEN FREE   SUPER EASY

Date paste is an excellent natural sweetener for cooking. You also can use it in place of jams or other fruit spreads. We use it to make our Sweet Potato Toast (page 12), Granola (page 32), and Carrot Nut Muffins (page 126).

2 cups packed pitted dates (about 16 ounces)

2 cups water

NOTE: To use date paste in your own recipes, substitute for granulated sugar in equal amounts (a 1:1 ratio). Note that in baked goods date paste tends to give a less chewy and more cakelike texture than granulated sugar.

VARIATION: When you're in a hurry or need only a small amount, use this method. The finished paste won't feel quite as smooth, but it takes just 5 minutes and yields ¼ cup of date paste.

½ cup pitted dates

½ cup very hot water (120–130°F)

1. Soak the dates in the water for 1 minute.

2. With back of a spoon, mash the dates gently in the water to soften them more.

3. Drain the dates, reserving the liquid.

4. Place the dates in a blender or food processor with 1 tablespoon of reserved liquid and process 15 to 30 seconds.

5. If needed, continue processing for a smoother texture, adding 1 to 2 tablespoons of the reserved liquid a little at a time.

---

1. Soak the dates in the water for at least 8 hours and as long as overnight.

2. Drain the dates, reserving the liquid.

3. Place the dates in a blender or food processor and puree.

4. Add a small amount of the reserved liquid and continue processing into a smooth paste. Add the liquid slowly as you process. You shouldn't need more than 1 to 2 tablespoons of reserved liquid.

5. Store in an airtight container in the refrigerator for up to 2 weeks.

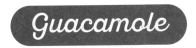

Guacamole

Yield: 3–4 servings | Prep Time: 7 minutes | Total Time: 7 minutes

FAST GLUTEN FREE GREAT SNACK SUPER EASY TASTER FAVORITE

We love the creamy goodness of guacamole as much for the taste as for the heart-healthy omega-3 fats. Enjoy this recipe as a dip, slather it on our Black Bean Burgers (page 52) or Burritos (page 55), or spoon it atop a salad in place of dressing.

2 large avocados

¼ cup finely minced onion

¼ cup finely minced tomato

1 tablespoon finely minced jalapeño or poblano peppers

⅛ teaspoon garlic powder

salt and pepper

1. Split the avocados in half or quarters and remove the pits.

2. To separate the flesh, slide a spoon between the avocado flesh and the peel and lift out.

3. In a medium bowl, mash the avocado flesh with a fork or potato masher.

4. Add the onion, tomato, peppers, and garlic powder and mix well.

5. Season to taste with salt and pepper and serve immediately.

> **TIP:** Guacamole is so easy to make for one or for a crowd. Allow approximately ¼ cup per serving, about half an avocado. For each avocado, add 1 or 2 table-spoons of the extra ingredients or to taste. If you're making for a gathering and it will sit out for a while, add 1 teaspoon lemon juice to prevent browning.

Panko Style Breadcrumbs

Yield: approximately 5 cups | Prep Time: 15 minutes | Cooking Time: 5–10 minutes | Total Time: 20–25 minutes

SUPER EASY

Homemade panko crumbs are easy to make and not terribly time consuming. Making your own saves money, and it's essential when you can't buy vegan panko locally and need them right away.

---

1 (16-ounce) loaf unsliced white bread

1. Preheat oven to 300°F.

2. Cut the loaf into 1-inch thick slices.

3. Remove the crusts and set aside.

4. Using a hand grater, grate the slices. You also can do this in a blender: Processing 2 to 3 slices at a time, pulse until the bread shreds into coarse crumbs.

5. On 2 large cookie or baking sheets, spread the crumbs in a thin layer.

6. Bake for 5 to 10 minutes. Fresh, moist bread may take longer, but make sure not to brown the crumbs.

7. Let the crumbs cool completely and store them in an airtight container.

NOTE: Your yield will vary depending on how closely you trim the crusts and how finely you grate the bread. In our testing, a 16-ounce loaf of white French bread yielded about 5 cups of panko crumbs, plus 1 cup of plain bread crumbs made from the leftover crust.

TIP: You can grate the bread in a food processor, but be *extremely* careful not to over-process. Use the metal chopping/mixing blade and process in small batches using only short pulses.

VARIATION: Don't waste those crusts! Turn them into plain breadcrumbs for use in fillings and coatings. For moist crumbs, pile trimmed crust into a food processor or blender and process thoroughly. For dry breadcrumbs, bake the crusts on a baking sheet at 300°F for about 10 minutes before processing.

Pickled Red Onions

Yield: 4 cups | Prep Time: 10 minutes | Cooking Time: 15 minutes | Total Time: 25 minutes

GLUTEN FREE   SUPER EASY

These onions might not be for everyone, but they do add a nice punch of flavor to sandwiches and salads. Try them on Black Bean Burgers (page 52) or the Chickenless Crispy Sandwich (page 28).

1–2 large red onions (to make 4 cups sliced)

1 (12-ounce) bottle red wine vinegar

1 teaspoon dried dill

½ teaspoon salt

1. Peel and thinly slice the red onions.

2. Place them in the air fryer baking pan.

3. In a small saucepan, stir together the vinegar, dill, and salt and bring to a boil.

4. Pour the boiling vinegar over the onion slices.

5. Cook at 390°F for 15 minutes.

6. Cool before serving and store unused onions in an airtight container in the refrigerator. These will keep for about 4 to 6 weeks.

See insert C7 for recipe photo.

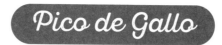

Pico de Gallo

Yield: 2¼ cups | Prep Time: 15 minutes | Total Time: 15 minutes

FAST   GLUTEN FREE   TASTER FAVORITE

Pico de Gallo is an excellent topping for quesadillas, enchiladas, or other Tex-Mex meals. We love it on the Burritos (page 55) and Calzones Tex-Mex (page 57). Add more or less jalapeño depending on how hot you like it.

¾ cup diced green or red bell pepper

2 tablespoons diced jalapeño peppers (optional)

¾ cup diced tomato

¾ cup diced onion

2 tablespoons lime juice

salt and pepper

1. In a medium bowl, mix together the peppers, tomato, and onion.

2. Stir in the lime juice.

3. Season with salt and pepper to taste.

Roasted Garlic

Yield: 1 pod | Prep Time: 5 minutes | Cooking Time: 15 minutes | Total Time: 20 minutes

GLUTEN FREE   SUPER EASY

Roast 1 garlic bulb or as many as your air fryer will hold in a single layer. You need only a tiny bit of oil, but if you prefer more, use our optional method below.

---

1 bulb garlic

1/8 teaspoon extra-light virgin olive oil

1. Preheat the air fryer to 360°F.

2. Cut off the top of the bulb to expose the tips of the cloves.

3. Drizzle the oil over the top of garlic clove tips.

4. Cook for 15 minutes or until the garlic softens and roasts through.

See insert C8 for recipe photo.

VARIATION: Use foil to hold the garlic upright so the oil soaks into the cloves instead of dripping into the bottom of the air fryer.

1. Preheat the air fryer to 360°F.

2. Cut off the top of the bulb to expose the tips of the cloves.

3. For each bulb you're cooking, cut a small piece of aluminum foil and shape it into a little cup around the bottom of the garlic.

4. Drizzle the oil over the top of garlic clove tips.

5. Cook for 15 minutes or until the garlic softens and roasts through.

Roasted Mini Peppers

Yield: 4–8 servings | Prep Time: 11 minutes | Cooking Time: 15 minutes | Total Time: 26 minutes

GLUTEN FREE   GREAT SNACK   SUPER EASY

Roasting brings out the natural sweetness in these little peppers, and they're so versatile that they're practically a staple at our houses. Try them in salads, sandwiches, sides, main dishes, stuffed with a filling, or plain for snacking.

1-pound bag mixed mini peppers, red, yellow, and orange

1 tablespoon olive oil

1. Wash the peppers, cut them in half lengthwise, and remove the seeds.

2. Toss them in oil to coat and place them in the air fryer basket.

3. Cook at 390°F for 5 minutes.

4. Shake the basket to redistribute the peppers and cook for 5 more minutes.

5. Shake the basket again and cook for another 5 minutes or until the edges of the peppers begin to brown.

Tex-Mex Seasoning

Yield: approximately ½ cup | Prep Time: 5 minutes | Total Time: 5 minutes

FAST   GLUTEN FREE   SUPER EASY

This salt-free seasoning will help you control the amount of sodium in a finished recipe. It tastes great in our Chickpeas (page 29), Pita Chips (page 37), Burritos (page 55), and Avocado Boats (page 80).

4 tablespoons chili powder

2 tablespoons onion powder

1 tablespoon garlic powder

1 tablespoon ground cumin

1 tablespoon oregano

1½ teaspoons black pepper

¼ teaspoon cayenne

Mix all ingredients together and store in an airtight container.

Texas Two-Step Dip

Yield: 6–8 servings | Prep Time: 5 minutes | Total Time: 5 minutes

FAST   GREAT SNACK   SUPER EASY   TASTER FAVORITE

We simplified a very popular regional dish to create a dip that's super-fast to make and still bursting with flavor. The Pita Chips (page 37) or Tortilla Strips (page 47) are excellent with this dip (assuming that you can resist eating it with a spoon!).

1 Roma tomato

½ red bell pepper

½ avocado

1 (15-ounce) can black beans

1 (15-ounce) can whole kernel white corn

3 tablespoons Italian salad dressing

1. Chop the tomato, bell pepper, and avocado. Then drain and rinse the beans and drain the corn.

2. Place all ingredients in a large bowl, stir to combine, and serve.

Tuscan Herb Mix

Yield: ¼ cup | Prep Time: 10 minutes | Total Time: 10 minutes

FAST   GLUTEN FREE   SUPER EASY

This salt-free seasoning elevates our Tuscan Tomato Toast (page 48) and Ratatouille (page 105).

3 tablespoons basil

2 tablespoons oregano

2 tablespoons rosemary

1½ teaspoons marjoram

1 tablespoon fennel seed

1 tablespoon garlic powder

1. In a food processer, add all ingredients and grind for 10 to 20 seconds.

2. Store in an airtight container.

JUST FOR FUN

E ating provides sustenance and necessary nutrients, but meals also should be enjoyable. The extra special and super easy suggestions that follow will make your special days even more special and ordinary weeknight meals extraordinary.

AFTERNOON TEA

Our Scottish Aunt Margaret once said that our Dundee Cake was as good as her mother's—the highest compliment! Invite 3 or 4 of your closest friends for book club or an afternoon of catching up. We like to serve a good Darjeeling, but we usually offer a variety of teas for our guests' enjoyment.

From the Recipe Index

Coconut Pound Cake (page 142)

Dundee Cake (page 143)

Creamy Chive Biscuits (page 132)

Cheddar Tea Biscuits (page 27)

Cranberry-Orange Scones (page 131) or
   Chocolate-Cherry Scones (page 127)

From the Store

1 hothouse cucumber (sealed in plastic)

1 loaf thin sandwich bread

strawberries, blackberries, grapes, or other easy-
   to-eat fruit

all-vegetable margarine or vegan butter

tea

nut milk(s) of choice

1. Make the cakes one day ahead. Cool, wrap, and set aside.

2. Earlier in the day, make the biscuits and scones.

3. Just before serving, thinly slice the cucumbers.

4. Spread margarine or vegan butter on the bread slices and top with cucumbers. These sandwiches look nice as open-faced sandwiches, but you'll find it neater to sandwich the cucumbers between two slices of bread.

5. Trim the crusts and cut the sandwiches in quarters.

6. Place the sandwich quarters on a pretty cake stand if you have one. Allow 4 to 6 quarters per guest.

7. When ready to serve, start the water to boil for tea and cut the cakes.

The Presentation

Use your prettiest dishes for serving and set everything out buffet-style. Let your guests help themselves. Serve sandwiches and savories first, then the scones, and lastly the cakes and other sweets.

GAME NIGHT

Our families love game nights, and they're great fun with friends as well. Here we offer a selection of easy-to-make and easy-to-eat treats with something to please everyone. These appetizers and snacks also make good selections for movie night. Organic sodas are a special treat for kids.

From the Recipe Index

Eggplant Fries with Curry Dip (page 31)

Spinach-Artichoke Dip (page 41)

Texas Two-Step Dip (page 160)

Mushrooms Stuffed (page 98)

Jalapeño-Tofu Sliders (page 34)

Tortilla Strips (page 47)

Guacamole (page 153)

From the Store

cookies

crackers

organic sodas

raw vegetables (baby carrots, cucumbers, bell pepper strips)

1. Earlier in the day, prepare the dips and sauce for the sliders. Pour into small bowls and refrigerate until ready to use.

2. Cook the Mushrooms Stuffed and set aside.

3. Prepare the tofu for the Sliders and cook.

4. While the tofu is cooking, prepare the Eggplant Fries, Tortilla Strips, and Guacamole.

The Presentation

Place the chips and crackers in separate bowls and set everything out buffet-style. If any of the food cools too much, you can reheat it in the air fryer easily.

ROMANTIC ITALIAN DINNER FOR TWO

Enjoy this meal alfresco with your special loved one. Set a table up on the patio or porch and dine under the moonlight. Start with a first course of Roasted Mini Peppers and Cheddar Olives. Chickenless Parmesan over angel hair pasta is our first choice for the main course with a mixed green salad on the side. You might prefer Mini Pizzas instead. Serve with a glass of Chianti Classico or Chianti Classico Riserva wine for an extra-special evening. Linger over a warm cup of espresso while gazing at the night sky.

From the Recipe Index

Roasted Mini Peppers (page 158)

Tomato Caprese Cups (page 46)

Cheddar Olive Nuggets (page 27) or Tuscan Tomato Toast (page 48)

Chickenless Parmesan (page 58) or Mini Pizzas (page 65)

Amaretto Poached Pears (page 135)

From the Store

mixed greens

mixed olives

grape tomatoes

salad dressing

espresso

vegan creamer

1. Earlier in the day, prepare the Mini Peppers and Cheddar Olive Nuggets. Both can sit out at room temperature for a few hours.

2. While the main course is cooking, mix the salad greens, olives, and tomatoes together. Just before serving, toss with dressing.

3. Prepare the espresso and add creamer to taste. Pour in an insulated carafe to keep warm.

4. Prepare the Amaretto Poached Pears.

The Presentation

Set candles on the table for a soft romantic glow and real cloth napkins. Prepare the plates in the kitchen and carry them to the table.

SUNDAY NIGHT DINNER

For many of us, Sunday nights are family time. Relax around the dining table and share your favorite memories of the week and weekend.

From the Recipe Index
Cherry-Berry Crisp (page 140)
Meatless Loaf (page 64)
Peas with Mushrooms & Tarragon (page 103)

From the Store
brown or white rice
nondairy frozen dessert (optional)

1. Earlier in the day, make the Cherry Berry Crisp and set aside.

2. Prepare the Meatless Loaf.

3. While the Loaf is cooking, cook the rice on the stovetop.

4. When the loaf finishes, remove it from the pan and set aside to rest while you prepare the Peas with Mushrooms & Tarragon.

The Presentation
In the center of a large shallow bowl or plate, mound the rice. Arrange slices of the Meatless Loaf around it and set the plate in the center of the table. Serve the peas in a separate bowl. For dessert, serve the Cherry Berry Crisp in small bowls and offer scoops of nondairy frozen dessert for those who want it.

SUPPER SOUTH OF THE BORDER

We live so close to the East Texas border that we might as well be Texans. We love Tex-Mex food and eat it often. We think you will love it too.

From the Recipe Index
Calzones Tex-Mex (page 57) or Burritos (page 55)
Tortilla Strips (page 47)
Pico de Gallo (page 156)
Guacamole (page 153)

From the Store
salsa

1. Prepare the Calzones or Burritos.
2. While they're cooking, prepare the Tortilla Strips, Pico de Gallo, and Guacamole.
3. Pour the salsa in a bowl and place it in the center of a serving platter.
4. Spread the Tortilla Strips around the outside of bowl.

The Presentation
Serve the Pico de Gallo in separate small bowls for each person. If your platter is large enough, place the bowls on the platter and surround them with the Calzones or Burritos.

AT-A-GLANCE RECIPE TABLE

Recipe	Fast	Gluten Free	Great Snack	Kid Friendly	Super Easy	Taster Favorite	Page
Breakfast & Brunch							
Breakfast Cornbread							2
Coconut Bacon	•				•	•	3
Donut Bites			•	•			4
English Muffin Breakfast Sandwich				•	•		5
Flourless Oat Muffins		•				•	6
Lemon-Blueberry Crepes	•		•			•	7
Oatmeal Bars	•	•			•		8
Peanut Butter Breakfast Sticks	•		•	•		•	9
Portabella Bacon		•				•	10
Strawberry Jam		•		•	•		11
Sweet Potato Toast	•	•	•		•		12
Taquitos & Jam		•					13
Toast, Plain & Simple	•		•		•		14
Veggie Sausage Corn Muffins						•	15
Appetizers & Snacks							
Artichoke Balls			•		•	•	18
Asparagus Fries			•			•	19
Avocado Fries	•		•			•	20
Avocado Taquitos		•	•				21
Banana Fries			•	•			22
Battered Cauliflower			•				23
Bell Pepper Rings			•			•	24
Cauliflower Spring Rolls with Peanut Sauce		•	•				25
Cereal Snack Mix	•		•	•	•		26
Cheddar-Olive Nuggets			•				27
Chickenless Crispy Sandwich			•		•		28
Chickpeas for Snacking		•	•		•		29
Chickpea–Sweet Potato Croquettes			•				30
Eggplant Fries with Curry Dip			•			•	31
Granola		•	•				32
Jalapeño Poppers			•				33
Jalapeño-Tofu Sliders			•				34
Mini Tacos		•	•		•		35
Pickled Okra Fries			•	•		•	36

Recipe	Fast	Gluten Free	Great Snack	Kid Friendly	Super Easy	Taster Favorite	Page
Appetizers & Snacks (cont.)							
Pita Chips	•		•		•		37
Potato Chips		•	•			•	38
Roasted Nuts	•	•	•		•		39
Smoky Sandwich	•		•		•	•	40
Spinach-Artichoke Dip		•	•		•		41
String Bean Fries			•				42
Stuffed Dates			•			•	43
Sweet Potato Fries		•	•	•	•		44
Texas Toothpicks			•			•	45
Tomato-Caprese Cups			•		•		46
Tortilla Strips	•	•	•		•		47
Tuscan Tomato Toast	•		•		•		48
Main Dishes							
Bell Peppers Stuffed with Hopping John		•				•	51
Black Bean Burgers		•					52
Bread Pockets							53
Brown Rice Bake		•			•	•	54
Burritos				•			55
Calzones							56
Calzones Tex-Mex							57
Chickenless Parmesan					•	•	58
Chiles Rellenos						•	59
Coconut Tofu						•	60
Empanadas							61
Fishless Sticks with Remoulade	•		•	•	•	•	62
Italian Pita Pockets							63
Meatless Loaf					•		64
Mini Pizzas			•	•			65
Mushroom-Onion Hand Pies							66
Pecan-Crusted Eggplant						•	67
Poblano Enchiladas		•				•	68
Polenta Half-Moons with Creole Sauce							69
Savory Corn Muffins				•			70
Seitan Nuggets			•				71
Sweet Potato Empanadas			•			•	72
Tofu in Hoisin Sauce							73
Tofu Sticks with Sweet & Sour Sauce							74
Vegetable Turnovers							75
Vegetables & Sides							
Asparagus Hot Pot	•				•		78
Asparagus Roasted	•	•			•		79
Avocado Boats	•	•			•		80

Recipe	Fast	Gluten Free	Great Snack	Kid Friendly	Super Easy	Taster Favorite	Page
Breads							
Artisan Loaf with Roasted Peppers & Olives							122
Biscuits			•	•		•	123
Blueberry Muffins				•			124
Bran Muffins							125
Carrot-Nut Muffins							126
Chocolate Cherry Scones				•			127
Cinnamon Biscuits				•		•	128
Cinnamon Pecan Bread							129
Cranberry Muffins						•	130
Cranberry-Orange Scones						•	131
Creamy Chive Biscuits						•	132
Tropical Muffins						•	133
Desserts							
Amaretto Poached Pears							135
Apple Pies				•		•	136
Apple Wedgies	•		•	•			137
Baked Apples		•		•			138
Banana Bread Pudding							139
Cherry-Berry Crisp		•	•			•	140
Chocolate Cake			•	•			141
Coconut Pound Cake with Pineapple-Lime topping						•	142
Dundee Cake							143
Gingerbread			•			•	144
Peach Fried Pies							145
Peach Pudding Cake							146
Peaches Poached in Raspberry Syrup		•				•	147
Strawberry Sauce		•		•	•		148
This & That							
Cajun Seasoning Mix	•	•			•		150
Croutons					•		151
Date Paste		•			•		152
Guacamole	•	•	•		•	•	153
Panko Style Breadcrumbs					•		154
Pickled Red Onions		•			•		155
Pico de Gallo	•	•			•	•	156
Roasted Garlic		•			•		157
Roasted Mini Peppers		•	•		•		158
Tex-Mex Seasoning	•	•			•		159
Texas Two-Step Dip	•		•		•	•	160
Tuscan Herb Mix	•	•			•		161

CONVERSION CHARTS

All values in these tables are approximate.

DRY INGREDIENTS BY WEIGHT

1 oz	=	1/16 lb	=	28.3 g
4 oz	=	1/4 lb	=	113 g
8 oz	=	1/2 lb	=	227 g
12 oz	=	3/4 lb	=	340 g
16 oz	=	1 lb	=	454 g

LIQUID INGREDIENTS BY VOLUME

1/4 tsp				=		1 ml
1/2 tsp				=		2 ml
1 tsp				=		5 ml
3 tsp	=	1 tbsp	=	1/2 fl oz	=	15 ml
		2 tbsp	= 1/8 cup	= 1 fl oz	=	30 ml
		4 tbsp	= 1/4 cup	= 2 fl oz	=	60 ml
		5 1/8 tbsp	= 1/3 cup	= 3 fl oz	=	80 ml
		8 tbsp	= 1/2 cup	= 4 fl oz	=	120 ml
		10 2/8 tbsp	= 2/3 cup	= 5 fl oz	=	160 ml
		12 tbsp	= 3/4 cup	= 6 fl oz	=	180 ml
		16 tbsp	= 1 cup	= 8 fl oz	=	240 ml
		1 pt	= 2 cups	= 16 fl oz	=	480 ml
		1 qt	= 4 cups	= 32 fl oz	=	960 ml
				33 fl oz	=	1000 ml= 1 L

FAHRENHEIT	CELSIUS
390	200
360	180
330	165
300	150
270	130
240	115
210	100
180	80
150	65

METRIC EQUIVALENTS FOR DIFFERENT TYPES OF INGREDIENTS

STANDARD CUP	FINE POWDER (e.g. flour)	GRAIN (e.g. rice)	GRANULAR (e.g. sugar)	LIQUID SOLIDS (e.g. butter)	LIQUID (e.g. milk)
3/4	105 g	113 g	143 g	150 g	180 ml
2/3	93 g	100 g	125 g	133 g	160 ml
1/2	70 g	75 g	95 g	100 g	120 ml
1/3	47 g	50 g	63 g	67 g	80 ml
1/4	35 g	38 g	48 g	50 g	60 ml
1/8	18 g	19 g	24 g	25 g	30 ml

For precise calculations, please see
http://www.metric-conversions.org/temperature/celsius-to-fahrenheit.htm
or check your preferred reference.

AIR FRYER BUYING GUIDE

A few short years ago, shopping for an air fryer was easy because so few models were available. Today, you have so many options that at first glance it can feel overwhelming. But finding the right model for you can be simpler than you might think. Air fryers are amazing little machines and not at all complicated. Before delving into details, your first considerations should be size and capacity.

Size

If you've never seen an air fryer, chances are that their size will surprise you. These are *not* small appliances. For many people, that's not an issue. It's a different story for those with tiny kitchens or efficiency apartments. When shopping online, pay attention to dimensions, including height. Do you have plenty of room on your countertop? Will it clear any overhanging cabinets?

Also consider ventilation. Most air fryers require some ventilation space behind, beside, and/or above the unit. You can find this information in the owner's manual, which should be available online. If not, look up the manufacturer's website and email or call them. If you can't locate a manufacturer website, consider another brand (more about that later).

Smoking shouldn't pose a big problem, but it does deserve some thought. Foods such as coconut can produce enough smoke to set off your kitchen smoke alarm, and so can a build-up of excess oil. For that reason, the best location for your air fryer is right next to your range so you can turn on the exhaust fan if needed.

Note that excessive smoking is *not* normal and may indicate that your appliance is malfunctioning. If that happens, safely disconnect power immediately and contact the manufacturer.

Capacity

It also may surprise you to discover that an appliance with such a large exterior has such a small cooking capacity. The two most common sizes are: 3.7 quarts (approximately), considered standard or regular size, and 5.8 quarts, the extra-large size. We designed all recipes in this cookbook for standard, 3.7-quart air fryers. This size is perfect for singles or couples but cooking for more than 2 people often will require cooking in batches. If you'll be cooking for 4 or more on a regular basis, definitely consider one of the extra-large models.

Features

Controls: Whether to choose manual or digital controls is strictly a personal preference. Neither option has significant advantages over the other. Some models offer presets that enable you to select a preprogrammed time and temperature by pushing a single button. It's a great idea, but it doesn't always work. Exact timing on any recipe can depend on how much food you're cooking, the temperature of the food when you begin cooking, and lots of other factors. Presets might be useful occasionally, but they aren't foolproof.

Timers: All air fryers have timers, but they don't all work the same. Some have a maximum setting of 30 minutes. That may accommodate most recipes, but foods such as large whole beets or casseroles cooked in a baking pan may require 40 minutes or longer. Timers also differ in how they function. Logically, when you pause your air fryer, you might expect a timer to stop, then continue from where it left off when you resume cooking. Most air fryers work that way but not all of them. On a few models, pausing the air fryer during cooking causes the timer to reset to zero. That means that each time you continue cooking you must reset the timer for the remaining time that you need. Another older but well-known model has a timer that can't be adjusted downward. If you accidentally set it for too many minutes, you can't reduce the time. You must wait for it to count down to the time you want and then start the air fryer. It's worth investigating specifically how a timer works before you decide which model to buy.

Accessories

To get the most from your air fryer, you definitely want to buy a baking pan. Breads and cakes turn out beautifully in an air fryer, and a baking pan

also enables you to cook mini casseroles, foods with sauces, and dishes with a high liquid content. You can use most any oven-safe dish, but a pan designed for the air fryer will have a handle. That makes a huge difference when you need to lift a pan of hot food from the basket without spilling it or burning yourself.

Some manufacturers offer a grill plate, usually sold separately. This plate has perforations and a ribbed surface that's more solid than the mesh air fryer basket. Such plates can be useful for getting a bit of a sear on foods such as pineapple slices, but don't expect the same results as with a traditional grill.

Another common accessory is the double-layer rack, used for cooking more food at once by stacking a second layer on the rack. It sounds good in theory but the problem is that during cooking you can't access the food on the bottom layer. To check for doneness, you must lift the hot rack from the basket without letting the food slide off. It's trickier than it sounds. Another issue is that in some air fryers the top rack sits so close to the heating elements that you can place only very thin foods there. Manufacturers include these racks with some models and also sell them separately.

Manufacturer and Warranty

Warranties on air fryers range from just 30 days to 1 year or longer, and terms can vary greatly. They may cover the unit, the parts, or both, and the coverage period for the parts may not align with that for the unit. Before you buy, look up the manufacturer's website. The owner's manual usually includes warranty information.

As mentioned above, if you can't locate a website for the manufacturer, beware. Who actually makes the product? If you buy it and have problems, who will help you? It's safe to assume that, if you have difficulty getting information from a company before the sale, you're not going to get any help from them afterward.

Price

Buying directly from a manufacturer almost always will cost you more, and it offers no advantages. Whether you shop online or at a local brick-and-mortar, make sure you choose a reputable seller. Before you buy, ask about their return policy so you'll know your options if something goes wrong. Even at the best companies, quality control isn't perfect. Besides, shipping can damage pretty much anything.

If you do have an issue, be sure you make the correct contact. The manufacturer usually handles warranty claims. To rectify problems such as shipping damage or receiving the wrong product, contact the seller.

For complete and up-to-date information on all air fryer brands and models, you can visit **TheHealthyKitchenShop.com**, which has charts to compare features side-by-side as well as detailed reviews of the top-selling air fryers on the market.

IMAGE CREDITS

INDEX